M000012731

FILL YOUR MIND

BEFORE YOU
FILL YOUR PLATE

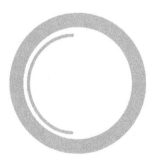

The Five Pillars Of Living
A Healthier Lifestyle

Faisal Alshawa

WRITING MATTERS

Fill Your Mind Before You Fill Your Plate

First published in September 2019

Writing Matters Publishing (UK)

ISBN 978-1-912774-38-8 (pbk)

ISBN 978-1-912774-39-5 (ebook)

Copyright 2019 Faisal Alshawa

The rights of Faisal Alshawa to be identified as the editor; and Contributors to be identified as contributing authors of this work have been asserted in accordance with Sections 77 and 78 of the Copyright Designs and Patents Act, 1988.

A CIP catalogue record for this book is available from the British Library.

All rights reserved. No part of this book may be reproduced in material (including photocopying or storing in any medium by electronic means and whether or not transiently or incidentally to some other use of this publication) without the written permission of the copyright holder except in accordance with the provisions of the Copyright, design and Patents Act 1988. Applications for the Copyright holders written permission to reproduce any part of this publication should be addressed to the publisher.

Disclaimer: *Fill Your Mind Before You Fill Your Plate* is intended as information and education purposes only. This book does not constitute specific health, medical, clinical, personal development or legal advice unique to your situation.

The views and opinions expressed in this book are those of the author and do not reflect those of the Publisher. The Author, Publisher and Resellers accept no responsibility for loss, damage or injury to persons or their belongings as a direct or indirect result of reading this book.

All people mentioned in case studies have been used with permission; and/or have had names, genders, industries and personal details altered to protect client confidentiality and privacy. Any resemblance to persons living or dead is purely coincidental.

Contents

7 At A Glance

9 Introduction

15 Section 1: It's All On You

17 Chapter 1: I Wish

21 Chapter 2: It Starts With The Self

27 Chapter 3: Go For It!

33 Chapter 4: Manage Your Environment

**37 Section 2: The Five Pillars To Living
A Healthier Lifestyle**

39 Pillar 1: Mindset

41 Chapter 5: Think Negative, But Stay Positive

45 Chapter 6: The Two A's: Anticipation
And Acceptance

51 Chapter 7: Old Mindset Vs. New Mindset

55 Chapter 8: Patience

61 Pillar 2: Belief

63 Chapter 9: Believe In Yourself

69 Chapter 10: Believe In Your Goals
And The Process

73 Pillar 3: Mindfulness

75 Chapter 11: Look Inwards

79 Chapter 12: Know The Voices In Your Head

83 Chapter 13: Emotional Eating

89 Chapter 14: A Mindful Mind

99 Chapter 15: Mindful Eating

107 Pillar 4: Sacrifice

109 Chapter 16: Organize Your Day Around
The Gym

113 Chapter 17: Endure The Pain

117 Chapter 18: Exercise Your Willpower

121 Pillar 5: Habits

123 Chapter 19: Fill Your Mind

127 Chapter 20: Break Those Habits
That Break You

133 Chapter 21: Take It One Habit At A Time

139 Chapter 22: Believe Nutrition Habits

145 Section 3: Nutrition For The Mind

147 Chapter 23: Sleep Hygiene

151 Chapter 24: Feed Your Brain

155 Chapter 25: Meditation And Nutrition

159 Chapter 26: Make A Healthy Lifestyle
A Part Of Your Life

163 Chapter 27: You Know Yourself Best

167 Section 4: Final Strategies And Steps

169 Chapter 28: The 7 Principles
Of A Healthy Lifestyle

173 Chapter 29: You Don't Have To Do It
On Your Own

177   Chapter 30: Choosing A Nutritionist

183   Chapter 31: Considering The Lifestyle Change

191   Chapter 32: Conclusion

195   References

197   About Faisal Alshawa

199   How To Get In Touch

At A Glance

Faisal Alshawa is a nutritional expert consulting to athletes and busy working professionals worldwide. His clients are typically successful people who recognise the need to make their health and living a healthier lifestyle a priority.

His first book, *Fill Your Mind Before You Fill Your Plate* is both a primer and impeccable gear change as well as a practical reference guide to creating and managing a healthy lifestyle ... starting with mindset.

Faisal Alshawa transformed his own health using the exact *Five Pillars For Living A Healthier Lifestyle* method outlined in this book, starting with a detailed exploration of the mindset required to making living a healthier lifestyle a life-long habit.

What makes this a highly readable reference is Alshawa candidly shares his own journey including the setbacks and struggles.

The Five Pillars For Living A Healthier Lifestyle are:

- Mindset
- Belief
- Mindfulness
- Sacrifice
- Habits

What makes *Fill Your Mind Before You Fill Your Plate* such an accessible read for anyone contemplating transforming their health, or for those looking for a mental edge to maintain a healthy lifestyle, is certainly the qualified insights, but also the open and conversational narrative.

Alshawa carefully describes his first exposure to a fitness culture as a Kuwaiti exchange student studying in the US. He then explains how he created a mental regime to stay on track.

That said, Alshawa is candid about the roadblocks, obstacles and setbacks he encountered and the ones you will encounter ... and should expect.

The chapters are clear and concise and this will drive your understanding, insights, application and momentum towards a healthier lifestyle.

Introduction

When I get asked by family and friends how I got into living a healthy lifestyle, I start by sharing my experiences as a student at the *University of Maryland*, College Park back in 2008. Even to this day, when I tell the story of my health journey, I always label myself as someone who was *sick in the head* during my transition into a healthier lifestyle.

What do I mean by this?

It was a time in my life where I was so focused, so dedicated and committed to living a healthier lifestyle, that it was sort of like an obsession—hence me being *sick in the head.* Some people might think this a good thing, others not. For me, it was a good thing.

During my journey, and mainly from 2009 – 2012, there wasn't a day that went by without me hitting the gym, whether to train or to recover from training. During midterms, on holiday, or even when I was feeling sick... there was always time for the gym because I made time for the gym. I had a goal and vision, and I was incredibly hungry to achieve them.

Today, I sit here writing this book running my own nutrition consultancy, *Believe Nutrition*, feeling in better shape than ever before. This is the first time I've ever put my story on paper, and writing all this now is giving me the chills because it really was one hell of a journey I went through. It was a beautiful journey, too, and a journey which turned me into the person I am today.

The question is, though, what got me to this point? How was I able to maintain exercising and eating well amidst the stress of university classes and other challenges presented to me at that time of my life? The answer is simple: the power of the mind.

See, wanting to live a healthier lifestyle is not only about healthy nutrition. It's not about training, either. It's a combination of both training and nutrition. However, even these two elements are not enough. Without the power of the mind, you won't get anywhere.

It all starts in the mind. Fill your mind before you fill your plate.

This book is about the five pillars that will help you live a healthier lifestyle. The five pillars are as follows, and in this order:

- Mindset
- Belief
- Mindfulness
- Sacrifice
- Habits

The advice I give you in this book is built purely from my own experience and knowledge gained from attaining degrees in Kinesiology (BSc) and Sports and Exercise

Science (MSc), as well as stories from my journey into building a healthy lifestyle and my experiences working with clients in my own business.

One thing you need to know before you continue reading on is that I was exactly like you.

When I first started my journey, I didn't have much support, nor the necessary level of education needed to know what to do and where to start. Even though I do specialize in the field of health and fitness now, as you read this book, you'll soon come to find out that I didn't start out studying in this field. So, what did I do then? Well, it was the change in my mindset that took me from *wishing* I could be like someone with a healthy lifestyle, or live in a certain way, to *actually* achieving it. But before I sought a gym membership, before I started reading articles on *bodybuilding.com* and asking *Dr. Google* what I should eat for breakfast, I looked within.

I focused on my mind.

This is the purpose of this book. I'm here to share my story, and to offer you my thoughts, feelings, and experiences in light of motivating and inspiring you to make the necessary changes in your own life. Just as I did with mine.

Transitioning into a healthy lifestyle, especially starting off alone, was certainly not easy. There were many good days, but there were also many days of doubt, discouragement, and shame, along with days where I simply lost self-confidence and belief in the possibility of me actually achieving the goal I had set for myself and the vision I had. But it was through lots of reflection and self-discovery that I was able to understand myself as well as my needs and wants in life. What's more? Developing the right mindset, self-belief, mindfulness, and a lot of sacrifice were pursuits that helped shape my habits and behaviors for the better. It was through this work, which I eventually developed into the *Five Pillars For Living a Healthier Lifestyle*, that I was able to become a healthier version of myself.

With all this being said, before you embark on your journey towards a healthy lifestyle, ask yourself *why*? Why do you want to live healthier? Why do you want to eat better? Why do you want to exercise? Determining your personal why will give you a true purpose and reason to live and achieve your goals.

As an example, when it comes to nutrition, it's important to differentiate between WHAT you're eating and WHY you're eating. If you go with the notion of what you're eating, you'll just eat or snack on whatever it is you're eating, be it healthy or unhealthy, without a real purpose. Maybe you're satisfying your sweet tooth, eating based off of emotions, or simply eating because you're hungry.

But when you know WHY you're eating, then you'll eat with a purpose.

You'll start to pay more attention to the foods you put into your body. You'll start to be more mindful and aware of your eating habits and behavior—all of which will help you eat healthier. It's the same thing for exercise and developing the right mindset. Why do you want to exercise? Why do you want to change your mentality?

Simon Sinek, author and motivational speaker, wrote a book that I absolutely love called *Start with Why*. In his book, he mentions a *Golden Circle* which consists of three parts: *why, how* and *what*. The *why* is at the center of the circle, followed by the *how* and then the *what* making up the outer portion. The *what* is something you can easily describe. It's what you do.

Keeping this relevant to health and fitness, it can simply be something like *I do Crossfit.*

The *how* explains the process and how you go about doing something. Sticking to *Crossfit,* perhaps this would entail you explaining your *workout of the day,* or your WOD as *Crossfitters* like to call it.

The *why* explains your purpose. Why are you doing *Crossfit?* The answer can be something like *I do Crossfit because I enjoy it and love the feeling I get after the workout.*

So, why start with the *why?*

As Sinek says, knowing your *why* gives you a reason and purpose to exist. Why do you want to live a healthy lifestyle? Why do you spend one hour of your day exercising? Or, why do you want to get to that point? Self-reflection and digging deep into your thoughts will help you understand this. You just need to spend some time thinking about it, and doing it!

What's my *why?* I want to be as healthy as I can for as long as I live. That means reducing my risk of illness as much as possible and being as independent as I can when I grow old.

My grandfather is a big inspiration of mine. To see him still swimming in the morning before going to the office every day at the age of 97 is truly something special. To see him being able to walk up and down the stairs and getting in and out of the car comfortably is something I aim to work towards.

On the flip side, I see other elderly individuals who are the complete opposite, and that makes me sad, to be honest. Put simply, I want to be as healthy and strong as possible, as I want to continue exercising and feeling and living well for as long as I live. This is what drives and motivates me every day.

This is my *why.*

So, before I start sharing my story, let me ask you this: *What's your why for wanting to be a healthier version of yourself?*

Take a moment to note down some of your thoughts.

_____

_____

_____

_____

Whenever you are feeling frustrated, unmotivated, or discouraged over not seeing results, or when any other obstacle (which I'll be describing in this book) gets in your way, always remember WHY you started. This is the reason why I want you to write it down. Revert to what you've written here whenever you need to in these situations—because remembering your *why* will allow you to bounce back, and not backwards.

Section 1

It's All On You

Chapter 1
I Wish

"If there's a single lesson in life,

it's that wishing doesn't make it so."

Lev Grossman

Let me take you back to May 31, 2008, my last day as a high school student at the *American School of Kuwait*. The journey had been long yet beautiful: coming into the school as a first grade student and remaining in the same school up until the twelfth grade. By that point, I knew what my fate was to include—continuing my studies by attending the *University of Maryland* (UMD) in the USA.

Why UMD? Well, aside from its gorgeous campus and reputable sports program, I wanted to live out of my comfort zone and be in a place where I knew absolutely no one. I had four years to spend in the US, and I wanted to make college a worthwhile experience, meeting new people and growing as an individual. What better way to grow than living out of your comfort zone, right?

Fast forward to September of 2008, my first month as a university student. The excitement was real. I moved into my dorm room, signed up for my classes, and got ready to kickstart my university journey. Unfortunately, being a freshman meant that I didn't have much priority when it came to picking the ideal times for my classes. I was left with a lot of early morning classes. In retrospect, this was a blessing in disguise.

There was one vivid morning that truly changed my life, and for the healthier. It was a Friday morning when my alarm went off for my 8am sociology lecture. I hated waking up at that hour to sit in a lecture! I don't know about you, but I'm the type of person who needs to get up at least two hours before any class or meeting in order to prepare myself and start the day on a calm note. On this Friday in particular, that meant getting up at 6am.

As I started getting ready for class, I glanced through the window of my dorm room and noticed men and women running on the streets of the university. This was so new to me. Coming from Kuwait, I'd barely seen anyone running at any time, let alone this early in the morning! While I was shocked to see this, I was also actually quite impressed, to say the least. It was hard enough to wake up at 6am to prepare for an 8am class. I couldn't imagine what it would be like to already be on the streets and running at six in the morning!

Growing up, I was never a *fit* guy per se. Sure, I was always into playing sports and doing some sort of physical activity, but I didn't necessarily have ripped abs and all. Eating healthy was something I did, but the awareness and amount of knowledge that was available back then was nowhere near what it is now. Sitting here writing this book, it's crazy to think about how much has changed in a span of over ten years. I always knew that exercise was key, and that eating well would make me live better, but not much more. Who should I blame, though? Was it the lack of general awareness at that time? Or was it the fact that I never really made a conscious decision to change my lifestyle for the better, and to make a healthy lifestyle a part of who I was?

So, going back to that moment in my dorm room, I thought to myself: *Man, I wish I had the motivation to get up at 6am and start running.* But, of course, like a lot of other thoughts in my mind, it was ignored while I just carried on with my day.

As I immersed myself more into the university and American culture, I realized how much time and energy people invested in fitness. The gym was always full of people, and I kept seeing students playing activities throughout the campus. Nine out of ten times, I would come across runners as I walked to my lectures. Why did I notice them so often? I wondered.... *Was it me feeling weird for not running, or was it people just being bored and having nothing better to do than running?*

Aside from noticing runners early in the morning, as months went by, I also started coming across the various athletes at the university more and more. Some were with me in the same classrooms, and others would be sitting at the table next to me in the dining hall. I was never surrounded by athletes, but I found myself being in awe of them, male and female! There were a couple of instances where I walked by football and basketball players, and noticed that they were huge! It was like nothing I'd seen before. Coming from Kuwait, I'd never once engaged with an athlete, so to be in a Division 1 sports university and see athletes like this was a new and exciting experience for me.

The level of athleticism I sensed just from looking at these athletes was unbelievable. After bumping into some of them and watching their games live, I would always tell myself, *I wish I had their physique* and *I wish I was as athletic as they are.*

Time went by, and before I knew it, I was entering my sophomore year. This was the year that everything changed. Having been in a new culture for a year, and immersing myself in an environment where health was prioritized, I thought to myself: *Enough wishing… I am going to start doing.*

From that year onwards, I put a goal in my mind, which was to simply *look* and *feel* like an athlete. I wanted to have the same muscular build as them, and to be able to share their same athletic qualities such as speed, agility, and coordination. I had a vision to be athletic, and I felt more ready than ever to start making that change.

Seeing those runners and athletes, I was sick and tired of wishing that I could be like them. While I knew I wouldn't ever be *exactly* like them—as we're all different, and there would be no way I'd attain the same athleticism they had—what I did know was that I could definitely gain the same drive and motivation to *feel* and *look* amazing.

If they could do it, why couldn't I do it? *I wish I could look like her. I wish I could train like him. I wish…. I wish.* People look a certain way, train in a certain way, and live a certain way for one reason only—*because of a decision they chose to make.* They became who they are by doing, not by contemplating, delaying, or postponing.

This is what I learned, and this is what I ended up doing. As a result, I'm proud to be where I am today.

Now it's your turn.

Chapter 2
It Starts With The Self

*"Without a humble but reasonable confidence
in your own powers, you cannot be successful or happy."*

Norman Vincent Peale

Self-Reflection

In 2008, when I moved to the US, I knew no one. That was the whole purpose of my move, though—to study at a university where no one knew me, and where I knew no one.

While I was anxious about living in a university only knowing a handful of people, it was actually a blessing in disguise because it helped kickstart my self-discovery journey. It's my university experience abroad that helped shape who I am today.

A big part of seeing success when trying to live a healthy lifestyle is based in relying on yourself. No one will make the choice for you to live healthier. The choice and decision all comes down to you. Since I had no family and only some friends, I needed to rely on myself for motivation and positivity. And if I wanted to rely on myself, I wasn't going to rely on an unmotivated, weak-hearted self. I wanted to rely on a strong and motivated self. Sure, I had the external motivation—like being surrounded by athletes and those who were already into health and fitness—but I needed internal motivation to keep going.

This is why I started to look inwards.

Luckily for me, living in a completely new environment meant that I had a lot of alone time. While it sucked to be alone at times, it was actually a great way to be able to start reflecting and discovering myself. Even if that meant sitting alone in the university mall in between classes, taking a walk at sunset to embrace the views, or simply sitting down in my dorm room for ten minutes and using no technology (whenever my roommate wasn't there), I tried to create some time for myself to reflect and think about who I currently was, who I wanted to be, and how I wanted to look.

So, why make time for yourself, you may wonder?

When you sit alone, you're able to sit down with your thoughts and really absorb everything. Even if it's just for ten minutes a day, that's a time when you can start reflecting on the type of person you want to be and the type of person you want to look like. But it's also an opportunity to connect with feelings, too. When you start thinking about the way you want to feel, it will start motivating you to start exercising and eating well in order to chase that goal and experience the feeling you put in your mind.

Think Of Your Future Self

So, being alone, I started thinking of my *future self*. I had a certain way I wanted to look, and I had a certain way I wanted to feel. Through connecting with all of this came the desire and the motivation I needed. I wanted to feel and look amazing, and the only way I was going to achieve that was to start hitting the gym and changing what I put on my plate.

When you're alone, you can start thinking about your *future self*. This element is so important, I can't emphasize it enough. You need to always be in touch with the person you want to be.

Do not treat that person as a stranger. Always connect with him/her because that will help keep you consistent and working towards your goals.

Transitioning into a healthy lifestyle is a journey. Just as I did, you're probably going to face a lot of ups and downs. Throughout the whole journey, and most importantly the downs, you have to always stay in touch with your *future self*. Always remind yourself of what you're trying to achieve and who you're trying to be. Period. It's only when you lose touch with this person that you'll start seeing signs of relapse. Stay connected, always.

Thinking of your *future self* doesn't necessarily mean thinking of yourself as having a six-pack. Absolutely not. But think of how you want your future to look like as you get older. Do you want to be able to live independently? Do you want to be able to live disease-free and injury-free? Do you want to be able to play actively with your kids and grandkids? These are the things that I'm referring to most. These are the things that I think about which continue to drive and motivate me to be the healthiest individual I can be. Think of your *future self often*. That person will thank you.

Find A Role Model

Growing up (and still today), I was always a football fan—otherwise known as soccer in some parts of the world, depending on where you live. Fortunately, during the start of my journey, I had someone to look up to. He goes by the name of Cristiano Ronaldo, and is arguably the best football player in the world.

To this day, he is a big inspiration of mine. Let me tell you why.

In 2004, I was lucky enough to watch Cristiano Ronaldo's *Manchester United* (my favorite football club) debut live at Old Trafford, *Man Utd's* home ground. At the time, he came off the bench and was unquestionably talented, but also a skinny, scrawny young boy.

I sit here today, as Ronaldo is scooping up a plethora of team and individual awards, having been nominated for the *FIFA Ballon D'or Player of the Year* award five times.

The amazing part of all this comes down to the fact that I've witnessed Cristiano Ronaldo's transition from a good football player to one of the greatest players the game has ever seen. Now, that's inspiring.

The time when I entered my *sick in the head* phase coincided with Ronaldo's rise to fame, finding his stardom status. So, luckily for me, his journey was happening at just the time when I needed the most motivation and inspiration. And what better way to get that rush of inspiration and drive than from none other than Ronaldo?

The point being, when you have a role model to look up to, you can learn from them and get inspired. Even if you're not there physically, when you see significant levels of growth, you can only conclude that it requires hard work, motivation, dedication, and commitment. These were some of Ronaldo's qualities that I admired and resonated with from the beginning.

Now, your role model might be someone completely different. No matter who it is, though, find that role model and get as much as you can from them. Believe me, this can be important. Sometimes, the frustration of self-discovery can accumulate and get you to start contemplating quitting, and even instill feelings of anxiety, anger, and stress. This is where the role model can come into play. Yes, self-reflection is important, but sometimes you just need that external motivation to give you a boost again and get you back on track.

I still have role models today. I was fortunate enough to have Cristiano Ronaldo to look up to during my transition phase. And you might have more than one role model, too. People like Kobe Bryant, and even someone completely out of the sports industry, Kendrick Lamar, are role models who I found myself looking up to later in my university days and who I still consider role models to this day. Believe me when I say that having people you can get inspired by will really help you in your journey. Especially when it comes to getting motivated from already motivated individuals.

So, who is your role model and how do you find them?

Well, for starters, your role model can be anyone who inspires and motivates you. This might be your grandfather, father, mother, any siblings you may have, or perhaps a friend whose work ethic, lifestyle, and personality inspire you.

It could also be a sports person, actor, or any other celebrity-status individual. It's very open-ended. The key, though—and this is how you should find them—is that such an individual should resonate with you and share the same values as you do. You have to admire some sort of characteristic of their personality; a characteristic that will allow you to become the best version of yourself.

The role model you choose should allow you to live with hope, determination, positivity, and belief in doing whatever it is you desire to do. They should serve as an individual who you can look up to as you keep striving and pushing yourself towards achieving your goals.

Chapter 3
Go For It

*"There's no reason to hold yourself back
and say you can't do something in life
unless you go for it and try to do it."*

Russell Westbrook

Okay, so I started the self-discovery process and was well into it. I'd go out to a beautiful lake near my university to go on runs, and when I got there, I'd do a few laps around the lake and then just sit there afterwards in peace, embracing the views and silence while I stretched. This was one way I paved the way for alone time and self-reflection.

Sometimes, I'd go out during sunset and sit by a canal right on the outskirts of the university. I loved being outdoors and surrounded by nature, so that sort of time made up a big part of my discovery journey.

To this day, I dedicate every Friday morning (which falls on a weekend back home) to exercising outdoors. I prioritize this time so much not only because of exercise and for the purpose of being outdoors, but as a means of simply disconnecting from everyone and enjoying my alone time training in a park (and not in a gym surrounded by people, which is where I usually exercise). It helps me absorb everything that has happened during the working week and also allows me to sit back and reflect on how I can improve myself the following week.

Another big part of my journey was trying different things—and I urge you to do that to understand yourself better. I took up music lessons (attempting to play the piano) while at university. I enrolled in a sound engineering course and learned how to use software for music production. I also learned how to DJ and started practicing that in my dorm room. In the case of exercise, I tried different classes and methods of training in order to figure out what type of exercise I truly enjoyed.

When you engage in different activities, your understanding of yourself and where your passion lies will slowly start to unfold. You'll realize what you like and what you don't like, as well as the things you are good at and not good at—all of which will help clear your mind and allow you to find a path that's right for you.

Let me share with you an example of a discovery I went through. It was during the second semester of my sophomore year when I realized the positive effects of self-reflection. Going into the University of Maryland, I'd enrolled as an economics major and begun working towards applying to the business school to study finance. At the time, I knew no better. Growing up in Kuwait, I was only exposed to majors like business, engineering, law, and medicine. Nothing else.

Anyway, as a prerequisite to applying for the business school, I had to start taking business classes. My first one was *Accounting 101*. I can't express to you enough how lost and unmotivated I felt during my first class. I felt so out of place that, literally, once the class was over, I went back to my dorm room and called my parents right away to express to them my feelings. There was absolutely no way I was going to continue with economics or apply to the business school. I just didn't relate to it, and had absolutely no interest in the class, let alone the field.

This was the point when I realized my self-reflection having some positive effects. I started to understand the things I wanted and didn't want. Thankfully, my parents were supportive, and the following year I double-majored with Kinesiology—the study of human movement. (Unfortunately, I couldn't drop economics as a major since I was on a scholarship specifically for that major, so having a second major was my only option.)

The discovery journey is never-ending, to be honest. It's a constant journey. But, as you understand yourself more and more, it gets easier with time, and what you've just read above about my studies shows only a slight example of how self-reflection can positively impact your life. When you start to understand yourself and do the things you want to do, the process will better allow you to live with purpose and intention. You'll start to be more confident in yourself and the decisions that are best for YOU and no one else. Such reflection helped me understand what I really wanted to do in life—to be involved in sports and exercise.

This is what led me to continue my studies by pursuing a Masters degree in sports and exercise science from *Loughborough University* in the UK, one of the top five sports science schools in the United Kingdom. It was what paved the way for me getting experience in working in football, something I'd dreamed about. I'd always wanted to be a football player, but once I realized that was not going to happen, I just wanted to be involved in the sport.

The alone time I experienced, the continuous self-reflection and discovery, allowed me to understand what I really wanted in life and where I wanted to go.

In the sense of living a healthier lifestyle, this self-reflection also made a big difference. On the occasions when my mind was telling me *not* to go to the gym, I was able to combat those feelings... *and go.* The awareness I gained also increased in relation to my diet, as I reflected on the way I ate, how much I ate, and what I ate. This allowed me to make healthier and wiser eating decisions. And I also made a group of friends who, fortunately for me, were also interested in exercising and going to the gym.

When you understand yourself more, you begin to have control over your thoughts and feelings. You start doing the things you enjoy (and avoiding things you don't), and surrounding yourself with people and places that push you forward.

Through these experiences, I started experiencing a greater sense of willpower. It was only when I was in the right mindset that I started to have the confidence to test my willpower. First and foremost, though, I had to honor my willpower. Just like I didn't want to rely on a weak individual during my phase of *being sick in the head*, I didn't want to promise something to myself and eventually break that promise. No, that wasn't going to happen.

So, when I wanted to experience a lifestyle and career change, I told myself to go for it, and to go all the way. I knew there were going to be setbacks, as with anything in life, but I had to overcome that somehow in order to keep going.

For example, in 2009 when I decided to make a career switch, I was really worried about what my future would look like. The health and fitness industry back home was nonexistent at the time, and I felt like I would have no career path after completing my studies. Battling the feelings of fear and doubt was a challenge, but I kept believing in myself and in my goals—I didn't want these negative feelings to get in the way. I grabbed any opportunity I had, worked for free a lot of the time, and did whatever I could to learn and get my foot in the door.

The question is, how did I overcome setbacks? This is where the idea of continually challenging myself comes in.

We all have this inner voice telling us what to do (or what not to do). We sometimes allow it to overcome our thoughts and emotions. See, I didn't want to have this voice take control of my thoughts, actions, and behaviors. I wanted to take over that voice. I wanted to take control and be the one in charge.

I had to stick to my promise and honor my willpower.

Self-reflect. Honor your will power. Challenge yourself. And then go for it.

Chapter 4
Manage Your Environment

"Choose to focus your time, energy and conversation around people who inspire you, support you and help you to grow you into your happiest, strongest, wisest self."

Karen Salmansohn

Don't underestimate the power of your surroundings. The people you're surrounded by and the environment you're in can play a big role in your progression towards a healthy lifestyle. Immerse yourself within positive energy circles and among those who will help support you on your journey. Believe me when I say this makes a huge difference! It certainly did when I was going through the transition.

Living in the US as a student in an amazing university, and being surrounded by a great fitness community, enabled me to stay motivated and committed to my goal.

I once watched Joe Rogan's podcast, *The Joe Rogan Experience*, when he hosted Kevin Hart. Literally, the first thing that Joe Rogan had to say was in regard to the fact that Kevin Hart and The Rock were two people who make him feel lazy the most (because they're so into their fitness routines). Kevin then mentioned how The Rock is an inspiration and motivation for him, and talked about the fact that it's good to surround yourself with those who inspire you and allow you to stay motivated to stay fit.

Here's what he had to say:

"He is a person that motivates me and inspires me. I think it's a blessing to be around that because it's truly uplifting. It just makes you weed out the circle. When you're around people that truly give you some good advice, serve a good value to your life, you then look at those who don't and you can then push them away. I'm big on personality. I'm big on energy. I'm big on will and wants. I believe that it is contagious. So, if you have a bunch of laziness around you… you're naturally just going to feed off [of it]. You're going to find yourself becoming what's in your environment."

I couldn't agree more with what he had to say.

From a nutrition point of view, managing your environment can definitely help better the way you eat. When you surround yourself with people who share the same goal as you in trying to be healthy, or are simply supportive and understanding of what you are trying to achieve, it will greatly and positively influence your ability to fulfill your health goals. You won't feel embarrassed when trying to eat healthy, and nor will you have to endure the pain and discomfort of being teased for trying to be healthy—something that can definitely slow you down in your journey.

I've actually had a lot of friends and family tease me along the way. It was hard to digest in the beginning. But then I thought to myself, *Why are people teasing me when I'm trying to do the right thing in taking care of my health and body? It should be ME who is teasing them for living a different lifestyle, not the other way around!*

When I thought of this, and got used to the teasing, I realized that I was doing the right thing by being on the healthy track. Ignoring the noise became easier, in fact, and the persistence and results I showed started to silence the critics.

You are increasing your chances for a successful lifestyle change when you manage your environment and observe potential pitfalls, including the influence of other people.

Here are some suggestions that may help you to manage your environment better:

- Surround yourself with those who inspire, motivate, and support you. If you are surrounded by negative people, always remind yourself of who and where you want to be. Remind yourself of the health goals you've set for yourself to allow yourself those priorities. Remember, you are the one doing the right thing by trying to be a healthier version of yourself.

- Be around positive energy, whether it comes from people, places, or things.

- Keep problem food (unhealthy food) out of sight.

- Avoid walking by vending machines if possible.

- Eat healthy foods in a structured meal plan. You won't be as hungry, which will help you manage cravings.

- If you are going to a beach house/chalet for the weekend, go grocery shopping beforehand to make sure you have healthy snacks and food available.

Sometimes it can be hard to take full control of your environment. Work may get in the way, and sometimes things like sweets and desserts may be lying on the table around your house. In the environment where you have no control, what are some things you can do to manage this? Here are some tips:

- Wait ten minutes before reaching out for that chocolate bar or bag of chips; don't go for it as soon as you consider it. Distract yourself with an activity—whether it's filing your nails, finishing one more work task, working on a crossword puzzle, or cleaning out the junk drawer. The craving may pass (really!).

- Try healthy swaps, such as snacking on baked rather than regular chips, dark chocolate instead of milk chocolate, protein bars rather than chocolate bars, and fruits instead of sweets.

- If meeting up with friends or family, perhaps eat beforehand or get a head start and look up the menu of the restaurant in order to plan what you will eat.

Section 2

The Five Pillars To Living A Healthier Lifestyle

Pillar 1: Mindset

Fill Your Mind Before You Fill Your Plate

Chapter 5
Think Negative, But Stay Positive

*"You're going to go through tough times - that's life.
But I say, 'Nothing happens to you, it happens for you.'
See the positive in negative events."*

Joel Osteen

Your journey towards a healthy lifestyle begins in the mind.

Living healthily is a long and non-linear journey. A lot of emotions are involved, both positive and negative. It requires a high level of commitment and dedication. It's going to take time and it will definitely be a difficult start. For those reasons, you need to start with a strong mindset, to be able to overcome the obstacles that come with trying to be healthy.

Compare your body to a strong building. Your mind is the foundation needed to keep everything else together. Changing your mindset isn't easy, but it's one of the most powerful things you can do to improve your life.

This is why *Mindset* is the first pillar.

Thankfully, I was able to develop the right mentality when I began to transition into a healthy lifestyle. Going to the gym six times a week, being careful of what I put on my plate, staying calm and collected—all these things required a lot of time and effort. I just kept telling myself to go forward and believing in the idea of hard working paying off.

Lazy days, soreness, pressure from balancing the gym with homework, exams, social events, travelling, days where my mind told me not to go to the gym or give into junk food…. These were things I kept thinking about.

It's these setbacks where you have to mentally train yourself if you're going to succeed, and you do this by putting the effort into doing things like resisting the temptations of eating unhealthy food, setting the alarm earlier to fit in time during the day to exercise, or eating a meal at home before going to a friend's house where you'll be surrounded by unhealthy food.

The positive moments, like when you finally see results, are the moments you should cherish and celebrate, but are not the moments that should take up the majority of your thoughts. Unfortunately, a lot of people tend to think of the positives when they get excited about turning their lifestyle around. I don't blame them, really. But then, once they get hit with the first obstacle, they don't know how to handle the situation because they haven't been anticipating it—and then they drop out and go back to square one. This is the part of the process that needs to be fixed.

The sad truth is, there will be many rough moments along the way, and if you're not mentally prepared to face those obstacles, you'll struggle to overcome them. On the flip side, if you think about the negative elements that come with living healthily, once they appear, you'll be better equipped to move past the situation successfully.

Here are some obstacles that my clients and I have faced in our own journeys, to give you an idea of what to prepare for:

- Fear of commitment

- Fear of missing out on good food

- Periods of no motivation

- Lack of patience (wanting to see results NOW, and wanting to drop out of a healthy program because no change has been seen)

- No time to cook meals or go grocery shopping

- Busy work schedules

- Social events (friends and family)

- Emotional eating

- Menstruation

- Feelings of laziness

- Consistency

- Easy access to food (like food delivery companies)

So, how do you overcome such obstacles? Anticipate and accept them. Normalise them.

When you are mentally prepared to face challenges along your health journey, and accept them, you'll be able to cope and overcome the challenge, and then continue carrying on along the healthy track. This sort of anticipation will allow you to keep tackling the challenges that come your way— because, believe me, they will keep coming.

The catch is that you'll only get stronger and stronger when facing these challenges, and hopefully, with time, they will be easier to overcome because you'll have mentally trained yourself to deal with such situations.

More on this in the next chapter.

Chapter 6
The Two A's: Anticipation
And Acceptance

"Acceptance doesn't mean resignation;
it means understanding that something is what it is
and that there's got to be a way through it"

Michael J. Fox

See, the first thing you have to do is recognize that it's going to be a bumpy ride. The second thing is to accept it. Be prepared for what's to come and just go with it. Prove to yourself that you can overcome these obstacles.

That's what I did. I *accepted* the slumps, but I told myself that, when I face any obstacle, I need to be strong and overcome the challenge. Defeat the obstacle. I didn't want the obstacle to defeat me and take me back to square one. This way, I was READY to face anything that was to come before me.

Let me give you an example. During the end of semester exams, I was anxious about a lot of things. How was I going to find the time to juggle studying, gatherings with friends, and the stress of exams, AND also now find time for the gym? It seemed like it just wasn't going to happen.

The first thing I decided to do was take a step back and envision the stressful times to come. Exam week was indeed one of the most stressful times for me. The key, though, was to realize the stressful times ahead of me and then prepare. So, I anticipated that things were about to get messy and I accepted it. I simply told myself that my life was going to be really stressful for the next week or two, and unfortunately I couldn't do anything about that because I did not want to fail my exams.

Simply anticipating and accepting the rough times brought a sense of calmness into my life, and I was able to think clearly and properly plan out my days—which is how I prepared for this phase of my life.

I'm a very visual and organized person, so I created a schedule of what subjects I'd be studying each day, the number of chapters I might have to read/review, and the number of hours I'd be dedicating towards studying per day (and I posted this schedule above the desk in my dorm room). Based off of this, I was then able to understand how much free time I'd have in any given day. Through my schedule, I realized the solution to effectively studying and also having time for myself was waking up earlier in the day. Doing so would allow me to study and finish my day earlier, to then be able to have the rest of the evening off for exercise. It was a double whammy, because I was also able to release the stress and pressure from studying at the gym—that was free time I made sure to have!

The plan worked smoothly. I accepted what was to come. I organized my time accordingly, and I was able to prioritize both studying and exercising.

The beautiful part of it all was that the exercise helped me stay more grounded during these hard times. It helped me release stress and also helped take my mind off of studying. I used to listen to my favorite playlists while smashing my workout at the gym. It was truly a great ending to the day. It was an awesome feeling to be able to keep this routine throughout out my midterms, and it worked. Maybe that's why I got good grades!

Nowadays, I'm self-employed and have many more responsibilities, so things are a bit different. What I do, though, is wake up early in the morning to get my work-out in before the day starts. I'll head to the gym, smash my workout, and feel more energized than ever before going to work. What's the best part of this? I come back home after a long working day, feeling tired and brain-dead, only to know that I have exercised and gotten that out of the way. I've been in those situations where I've promised myself I'll go to the gym after work, and it never happens. It's not a nice feeling, either—especially if it happens more than once during the week.

I accepted the fact that work will consume my day, and may leave my feeling tired and lethargic. I was prepared for this, as I've also been in those situations before. Seeing as I already knew this and accepted it, when the time came, I was able to get into the habit of hitting the gym in the morning so as not to face any workout obstacles throughout the day.

Now I have my own business and face plenty of different stresses in life. Long working days, presentations, interviews, meetings, you name it! How do I cope with these stresses?

Over time, I realized the plan of waking up earlier in the day did wonders for me. I did not mind it at all; it suited my lifestyle and it felt right. It was something I was able to do consistently, too, which was the key to its success. To this day, I wake up early in order to make sure I can fit in as much as possible during the day, and will actually wake up earlier if I anticipate having a long working day or stressful week. The only difference is that I'll exercise in the morning rather than the evening.

So, what about you? How can you cope with the stresses of work, for example?

Let's say you're an employee at a company that's outside your own control; the good thing is that you'll already have an understanding of what your working week will look like. You may have a presentation lined up (to give or attend) or have lots of meetings scheduled. Given this, you already have the anticipation element nailed down. You'll most likely know the working week ahead, so you just have to accept it—there's nothing you can do about it unless you want to skip out on everything and get fired! When looking at your workweek and planning ahead, the idea of meal planning is an excellent thing to embrace and implement. Going to the grocery store over the weekend and preparing your meals for the week can do you wonders in staying on the healthy track.

How do you meal prep? Sometimes, the hardest part of meal prepping is getting started. If you're new to meal prepping, here are my best tips for starting off on the right foot:

1. Start small with two- or three-ingredient recipes until you get the hang of it.

2. Cook in batches. For example, grill several chicken breasts that may last you for 2-3 meals.

3. Keep it simple and stick to recipes you know and love.

4. Don't give up! If you don't like your meals one week, switch it up and try again next week.

I'll be honest and tell you that meal prepping can be a tedious task, especially in the beginning. But at the end of the day, it's the best way to keep you on the healthy track since you are in control of your portions, the ingredients you add, and the way you cook your food!

Chapter 7
Old Mindset vs. New Mindset

"Mind is a flexible mirror.
Adjust it, to see a better world."

Amit Ray

We all have our ways of doing things. We also have different perceptions. Usually, what happens is that over time you get used to living a certain way. You end up thinking a certain way which dictates you living a certain way. This is just who you are. This is the way your mind works.

Now, start challenging your mindset with a new stimulus, a new way of doing things. You might accept such new stuff at first, but what usually ends up happening with most of us (and again, this is something I've experienced) is that our old mindset takes over. We're just so used to doing a particular thing or thinking a certain way that we'll find it very hard to challenge ourselves with a new stimulus.

Let me give you an example. You have a cake in front of you. Thoughts start rushing in your mind. *Should I have a slice? Should I not have a slice? One piece won't really ruin my workout today. Will I put on weight if I eat cake?*

We've all been there, right?

So, what do you do?

You reach for the cake and cut yourself a slice. Fine— if this happens one time, no biggie at all. But then you're invited to your family's house the week after that, and there you see cookies being put on the table after lunch. You get into the same cycle again. Your mind starts going all over the place for a few seconds, but then you eventually reach for the cookie.

You experience this a third time, and then you give in. A fourth time, and then you give in, again and again. You can see the pattern here. With time, especially when you keep giving in to the dessert and not challenging yourself via the other thoughts which are telling you NOT to reach for the dessert, your mind just gets so used to giving in all the time. It will become ingrained in you. Sure, there may be some times where you can resist, but the majority of the time, you'll give in.

When it comes to wanting to live a healthy lifestyle, you can't let your old mindset dominate you. You'll never grow if you do. You've got to fight the feeling. You have to let the other thoughts take over—the thoughts holding you back from a craving, that can start letting this new mindset be the dominant force. Because only when it's the dominant force will you be able to resist the temptations of always reaching for a dessert after a meal.

This is just a slight example that I feel you can relate to because we've all been there before. With me, when I first started, I kept fighting through it. Even if it meant going through the short yet powerful mental stress of deciding whether to reach for the dessert, eat unhealthy food, or get to the gym. But I knew that if I just sucked it up for the first month or so, I'd eventually get into the routine of my new way of doing things. I'd allow this new mindset to overcome my old mindset.

While I went through a lot of resistance and emotions, today I find myself not having many temptations, and when I do face them, I'm able to handle it much better than I used to. This is a rewarding feeling; it really is. Because even if I do give in during one meal, or even for a whole day, I know that because this mindset is now ingrained in me, I can go back to the gym the next day and eat healthy meals all over again—living healthy is my new norm, but it took work and breaking that old mindset to get here.

Having said all this, my advice to you when trying to start living a healthier lifestyle is to fight your current (and old) mindset as much as you can. Try to resist the thoughts telling you to eat that cake, or skip the gym, or to eat more.

You need to first understand that adopting a new mindset will be challenging, but you have to know that this only happens in the start and will get better—if and only if you allow the new mindset to govern your mind fully. The more you absorb a new mindset, the more you'll be able to dominate your old one.

This will make a strong and positive mindset a part of you. Believe me when I say that, when this happens, you'll feel like you can take on anything. You can resist temptations much easier and without lots of stress, you can allow yourself to keep exercising, and you'll find yourself making decisions that are healthier for you. Ignore the voice saying, *I can't.*

Change the way you think. Redefine the way you live.

Chapter 8
Patience

"Patience and perseverance have a magical effect before which difficulties disappear and obstacles vanish"

John Quincy Adams

Throughout my journey to a healthy lifestyle, there were many moments where I thought to myself, *Man, when am I going to start seeing results? Is this hard work all for nothing?*

As I started to read more and more articles on the internet and got to know a bit more about the physiological responses in the body, I came to realize that time was required for physical results to actually start showing themselves. Especially for me, given my body type and genes.

Weightlifting was the main form of activity I did in the gym. Not to get too scientific on you, but it came to my attention that the first signs of improvement that are typically seen with weightlifting are neuromuscular. This means that motor neurons, nerve cells, can more effectively send signals from the brain to the muscles. This in turn will enhance the recruitment of muscle fibers to contract and produce force. In other words, the connection between your brain and muscles will get stronger; hence, your muscles will experience stronger contractions to improve things like muscle growth, strength, and power.

So, I thought to myself: *Okay, let me keep going and not get discouraged. Clearly, this is going to take time, but the more I lift weights, the more I'll improve my neuromuscular activity, and the closer I'll get to seeing physical results.*

It's a journey, indeed. Nothing is going to happen over-night, and that is what I came to learn. Patience is a virtue in life in general, and it's also a virtue when it comes to stay-ing strong in your journey towards a healthier lifestyle. Look, all the elements within developing a strong mindset are important, but I can't stress to you enough how important patience is!

Believe it or not, I've had the occasional client sign up with me for a three-month nutrition program and literally drop out just two weeks into it. I take weekly body weight measure-ments as a means to monitoring my clients' progress. After the second measurement, which showed no improvement to the first bodyweight reading, one client dropped out because she was expecting results already—by the SECOND week!

These are individuals who not only ignored the obstacles that they were going to face in their weight loss journey, but also ignored the time it would take to see results. They did not accept it. Their old mindset (*expecting to see rapid results*) was not challenged by the new thoughts I was trying to ingrain in their minds (*patience*). As I discussed in the previous chapter, this client's current/old mindset dominated the new mindset, which led to relapse. She didn't acknowl-edge the obstacles, and she didn't accept the new mindset, so she continued to be impatient, which led to decreasing motivation levels and going back to square one.

Understand that achieving your goals, whatever they may be, requires time. So, be patient. In your professional career, you have to be patient, right? You're not going to be a CEO from day one. In your athletic career, you're not going to be considered the best at your sport from day one. Likewise, in your healthy lifestyle journey, you're not going to be healthy and lean from day one, either. I'm sorry to burst your bubble if that's news, but it's simply not going to happen.

So...

Take Baby Steps

Let me tell you a secret of mine. Something that allowed me to be patient throughout my own journey. My goal in the beginning was to gain muscle mass. I didn't want to have that body-building type of look, but I definitely wanted to gain more muscle. Now, given my somewhat scrawny figure at the time, if I'd immediately envisioned myself being big without putting in the work, time, and effort needed to get there, I would've dropped out after the first month. Because getting big (and achieving any other goal, for that matter) requires time.

So, instead of thinking about the end result, which was always at the back of my mind—to keep me grounded and remind myself of the bigger goal I was trying to fulfill—I broke down my goal into smaller steps. I took things step by step.

For instance, I broke it down into three-month intervals. I told myself that I would take girth measurements every three months, especially around my arms and chest, to monitor my growth, but also to make sure I hit certain targets. Of course, hitting the small goals was not easy, but it made things much more realistic and allowed me to exercise my patience much better than if I'd thought about achieving my bigger goal from the get-go! Taking things step by step, three-month interval by three-month interval, I eventually hit my bigger goal.

This is my recommendation to you.

If you want to achieve a certain goal, break it up into smaller incremental milestones. This way, you can stay patient while still maintaining the work, and, if anything, increasing your motivation levels to then help you achieve the bigger goal.

Let me give you a good example of a common goal: weight loss.

Let's say your goal is to lose 10kgs. If you're hung up on the number 10, you won't get anywhere. To make it a smoother and more exciting journey, break up your total weight loss target into smaller targets—let's say 2kgs per milestone.

The recommended weight loss to be experienced on a weekly basis is anywhere between 0.5kg – 1kg. Although some individuals may experience the loss of 4kg of weight in one month, others may find this more unrealistic and difficult to accomplish. Two kilograms in one month is very doable and realistic. With that being said, aim to lose 2kgs per month. Yes, this may mean your larger goal will take five months to accomplish, but trust me, it helps you stay in the game for much longer while helping you stay sane, patient, and motivated throughout your weight loss journey.

You get my point here.

Many people are impatient to reach their goals because they only think about the end goal. They don't think about the journey (or process) it takes to get there. They don't understand that it requires time, hard work, effort, and dedication. So, predictably they relapse. Whereas, if you take your bigger goal and break it up into smaller parts, and go about your journey in baby steps, believe me when I say you'll fulfill your goal.

And you'll be the happiest person when you do so.

Pillar 2: Belief

Chapter 9
Believe In Yourself

*"Believe in yourself, and the rest will fall into place.
Have faith in your own abilities, work hard,
and there is nothing you cannot accomplish."*

Brad Henry

What if everything you *thought* you knew about your health was wrong?

What if your health is, actually, nothing more and nothing less than what you *believe* it to be?

Your beliefs have consequences. Look at the *placebo effect.* If you *believe* a tablet will help you, then *help you* it likely will. The opposite is no different. You need to change the way you think and believe that you already have the things you want. Say to yourself: I am *already* healthy. I am *already* strong, resilient, and free from pain. Positive expectations have a positive impact, and your beliefs are directly linked to your health.

Indeed, once you've developed a strong and positive mindset, the next thing you need to do is start believing.

There are lots of things you can believe in, but first and foremost is the need to believe in yourself. You're the only one that has control over your life; no one else. Your decision to transition into a healthy lifestyle should be your decision. To make that decision, you have to believe in yourself. You have to believe in your potential to make you go through the transition successfully and allow you to reach your goals.

Funnily enough, I'm a huge believer in the word believe. It's true, though. Once you believe in the power of the word, it can take you a long way. It makes you feel confident, strong, and in charge of your own life.

I remember the word really resonated with me back in 2008 during the semi-final round of the *UEFA Champions League*, a huge tournament between the top football clubs in Europe. It was *Manchester United vs. Barcelona* at Old Trafford, and the club pre-arranged for one section of the stands to spell out the word *BELIEVE*. They did this by putting colored paper accordingly on every seat across the stands to then be lifted up when the teams walked through the dug-out tunnel and onto the football pitch.

The moment I saw that, I got goosebumps. In fact, *Manchester United* won that game and went on to win the whole tournament, with the word *BELIEVE* being displayed once again in the final! Me being a 17-year-old football fanatic at the time, seeing that word shown on such occasions and to also see my team winning made me think of how powerful a word can actually be. I really am blessed and thankful to have witnessed such a thing because it truly created a positive association with the word, and I've kept that with me. I'll always believe.

But this book isn't about me. It's about you. The fact of the matter is, *you* have to believe in yourself. A lot of us may think that our personality, beliefs, intelligence, and physical abilities are limited. We may think that no matter what we do, we will never improve. Because of that, we tend to focus on doing things to prove to ourselves that we can achieve them, not because we genuinely want to change and develop.

Some of you reading this may already have heard of the terms *fixed mindset* and *growth mindset*. If you haven't, let me just briefly explain them to you. A *fixed mindset* is when a person believes that their abilities and qualities do not change; they're fixed, as the word suggests. On the other hand, those with a *growth mindset* are individuals who believe that their abilities and qualities can be cultivated and grow and develop with time and experience.

How do you know which mindset you have and how to transition from one to another?

Let me give you an example of someone with a *fixed mindset* in terms of weight loss. An individual with a *fixed mindset* believes they either can or cannot lose weight. There is no in between, and there is no belief in going through the process of learning and improving themselves. People with this mindset towards weight loss will then put up barriers between them and any uncomfortable situation (like going to the gym, or pushing themselves during exercise) and feel like they are useless.

Furthermore, if they mess up, such as with eating junk food or having a slice of cake, they'll put themselves down and simply say *I can't do this*. Small slip-ups will keep them feeling frustrated with their actions and self. Individuals with a *fixed mindset* may go on crash diets (restricting themselves from food) to lose a certain amount of weight in a certain period of time, not knowing what the consequences will be after that. They just want to focus on the number on the scale without thinking about other factors affecting their lifestyle.

On the other hand, someone with a *growth mindset* will understand that effort is needed in order to see success, and believe it is possible. If they are trying to lose weight, they'll know that, with time and effort, they'll be able to master their nutrition. Those with a *growth mindset* will take things day by day, focusing on the process and making healthy and smart choices. They'll have a goal to work towards, but they won't focus on only the outcome. In a case where they mess up, as in the example above, those with a *growth mindset* will learn from their setbacks and improve themselves— hopefully not repeating the same mistake again.

In the case of living a healthier lifestyle, those with a *growth mindset* will focus on their lifestyle and how to improve themselves on a daily basis. They won't focus on fad or celebrity-endorsed diets. Rather, they'll be eager and curious to know how they can make adjustments to their lifestyle in order to simply eat healthier, move more, and make better and healthier decisions on a daily basis. Their ultimate goal is to be a healthier and happier version of themselves, regardless of how they look or the number on the scale.

Which mindset do you have? It's a no-brainer that you must have a growth mindset to not only transition into a healthy lifestyle, but to sustain one as well.

This didn't happen overnight for me, and nor did it come easily. It came with time, effort, consistency, and genuinely believing in myself. After all, your mindset is shaped by your beliefs and attitudes. If you believe yourself to be one with a *fixed mindset*, or are looking to change your old way of thinking, now would be the time to start working towards having a *growth mindset.*

So, how can you develop a *growth mindset?* Here's what you can do:

- **Embrace a challenge.** As I've mentioned, you will be facing challenges along your health journey. Embrace these challenges, and use them as opportunities to learn more about yourself and how you can improve.

- **Accept the journey.** I've already discussed this, but it matters here; when you accept that you will experience challenges, you can start making small changes in your lifestyle that will help you overcome such challenges.

- **Find what works best for you.** The way I cope with challenges may not be suitable for you, and vice versa. Find ways that are convenient for you to make small changes to improve your lifestyle.

- **Focus on the process.** You may be the type of person who cares a lot about your weight. Rather than focusing on that, though, focus on the process to reach your desired weight.

- **Continue to learn.** Always take something out of the challenges you go through. Use them as learning experiences. Through learning, you won't repeat the same mistake twice.

- **Remember your *why*.** This is a good time to look back at your *why*. Remember why you are starting on this journey, as this will give you a sense of purpose which will help you develop such a mindset.

My advice to you is this: embrace the fact that you can change and become a healthier version of yourself. As you'll come to find out in Chapter 19, you can rewire your brain and develop a new mindset. It's scientifically proven!

If you do this, you will make better choices and reach your full potential. Believe in yourself.

Believe.

Chapter 10
Believe In Your Goals And The Process

"You control your future, your destiny.
What you think about comes about. By recording
your dreams and goals on paper, you set in motion
the process of becoming the person you most want to be.
Put your future in good hands - your own"

Mark Victor Hansen

When I started to believe in myself, I automatically started to gain more self-confidence. With belief and confidence, I was then able to start believing in my goals and work towards them to start achieving.

After believing in yourself comes believing in your goals. You should never be in a situation in your life where you set forth a goal without believing you can actually achieve it. The same applies when you're setting up your health goals. For me, it just does not make sense to set myself a goal and not believe in it. Whether you achieve this goal or not comes down to a lot of factors, but you most certainly need to believe in yourself and your goals when you place them.

Be SMART With Your Goals

Through my own personal experience and also experience working with clients, I've come to realize that some people tend to set unrealistic goals. But setting unrealistic goals itself creates feelings of disbelief. When you don't achieve the goal, you'll feel even more frustrated, and doubt yourself even more when it comes to the possibility of achieving future goals.

This is why it's key to set SMART goals when starting your journey to a healthier lifestyle:

- S: Specific

- M: Measurable

- A: Attainable

- R: Realistic

- T: Timely

Let's use an example of someone who wants to lose 10kg in five months. It's important to have the number ten in the back of their mind, but it shouldn't be the main number to focus on. As I mentioned earlier, healthy weight loss is considered to be anywhere between 0.5kg to 1kg per week—this to lose weight in the right way without gaining it all back easily. That means someone may lose 2-4kgs per month. So, rather than focusing on 10kgs, take things week by week and focus on losing 0.5kg to 1kg per week.

Notice here that the goal is first specific—losing 10kgs in five months. It's measurable, because one can check their body weight each week, and also aim for 0.5kg to 1kg weight loss per week.

It's most certainly attainable, because losing 2-4kg per month is not incredibly difficult if you put your mind to it. Losing 10kgs is very realistic in this time-frame, and five months is a good enough cushion to account for any roadblocks along the way that may hold them back from moving forward, while also providing enough time to overcome such roadblocks and still achieve the set goal.

So, please, the next time you set a goal for yourself, whether it be weight loss, weight gain or any other type of goal, make sure it is SMART. When you strategically map out your goal-setting plan, you'll feel more confident and comfortable with yourself and your goal; as a result, you'll most certainly have the belief in yourself to achieve the goal at hand.

Believe In The Process

If you believe in yourself and in your goals, now you have to believe in the process. When I first told myself that I wanted to become a healthier and better version of myself, I knew that it wasn't going to come easy, nor overnight. I told myself that it was going to be a process. If I focused only on the future person I wanted to look like and feel like, I would have felt depressed because I'd know that it would be hard to achieve that goal. I'd feel bummed out and start to lose belief in my goal, let alone sustaining any self-belief.

Thankfully, that didn't happen. I was fortunate enough to realize and understand the fact that this transition would take time, effort, and patience. I was able to break up my journey into parts and take everything day-by-day, month-by-month, and year-by-year. And it worked well for me.

If you talk to any other health and fitness professional,

they'll most likely give you the same advice as I will. That is, to believe in the process and take the baby-step approach. If you have a specific goal in mind, don't think of the end goal. Yes, have it in the back of your mind, because that's the goal you want to end up achieving, but don't make it the main focus because doing that really could backfire. It could make you feel sad and anxious, and eventually lead you to drop out from the process entirely.

Continuing with the simple example above, if the person who wanted to lose 10kgs only focused on that number, they would feel a bit anxious because it's not a small amount of weight to lose, especially if they wanted to lose weight in a short period of time.

However, if that person believed it was going to be a process and journey to lose 10kgs, and compartmentalized the big goal into smaller goals, they would have a more pleasant time achieving their goal. They'd also find it to be a much smoother journey.

Taking all this into consideration, they would have a greater ability to reach their goal and have more fun while doing so. The fun would then lead to consistency, and the consistency would lead to achieving more frequent, smaller goals on the path to reaching the end goal.

This is the way I achieved my health goals, and this is the way I recommend you do so, as well.

Believe.

Pillar 3: Mindfulness

Chapter 11
Look Inwards

"It's the inward attention that takes you into the depth of the mind."

Roshan Sharma

According to *Cambridge Dictionary, mindfulness* is *the practice of being aware of your body, mind and feelings in the present moment, thought to create a feeling of calm.*

For me, mindfulness comes in many forms. You need to be mindful with your emotions—knowing how to control your own thoughts to then elicit desired behaviors and actions. When it comes to training and exercise, you also need to stay mindful, and all the more so when it comes to training in the zone and staying focused. Even when you eat, you need to eat mindfully at every meal by not only being aware of what you put into your body, but how you eat, as well.

Indeed, you need to try as best you can to be present in the moment throughout your journey to a healthier lifestyle. As I alluded to in previous chapters, making the transition is not easy. Stress, anxiety, doubt, and fear are all emotions that you'll most certainly experience at some point in your journey. I'd be lying if I told you that you won't experience any negative thoughts and emotions.

With mindfulness, you'll be able to look inwards and recognize these negative thoughts and emotions. In fact, that's the first step—to be mindful or aware of such triggers. Like everything else I've described so far, practicing mindfulness is also not easy and definitely requires time. Let me give you the slightest of examples as to what I mean regarding being aware of a trigger. Imagine yourself driving to work on a nice, sunny day. Music is playing in the background and you're feeling good, but then, suddenly, another car cuts in front of you. What's your natural response? You start road-raging and honking your horn uncontrollably. You might very well find yourself cursing the driver!

This kind of reaction is the second nature reaction.

It's the reaction undergone when being *mindless*. Now, let me give you an example of how a mindful person might react. As soon as the other car cuts in front of them, they may get the urge to scream their lungs out, but instead, they just take several deep breaths and avoid letting that stupid driver get to them. Rather, they'll continue to enjoy driving through the beautiful weather, listening to the music playing and enjoying the good vibes.

This is just the most basic example, but it's a good one since some of us experience this on an everyday basis, if not multiple times a day!

In the case of nutrition, we all go through different stresses during the day.

Let's say you had an extremely stressful working day and are fed up with some of your colleagues. To relieve the stress at work, you end up reaching for that basket of chocolates, or perhaps a jar of pretzels, and start munching like crazy. Before you know it, you've consumed so much sugar, or 500 calories worth of pretzels, and then feel really guilty and frustrated with yourself. That is *mindless* eating.

Now, on the other hand, what if you took a step back when you were feeling stressed and just checked in with yourself for five minutes? You could take a deep breath and ask yourself, *How am I feeling? Am I actually hungry or just stressed out and emotionally hungry?*

I like to call this *taking five*—meaning, taking five minutes of your time to check in with yourself before delving into the bowl of chocolates in your office. By doing that, you are being *mindful*. You are aware of your stress and the situation at hand, and making an effort to take five minutes out of your time to understand your feelings and emotions before diving into food to comfort yourself.

Notice that you are *noticing.*

Believe me, being mindful is an extremely important characteristic that you must adopt throughout your journey, and in life in general, too.

That's why it's one of the *Five Pillars.*

Chapter 12
Know The Voices In Your Head

"We must carefully cultivate the voice that speaks to us
because an internal voice is the ultimate narrator
of our charming and delightful personal story
or the documentarian of our tragic
and disgraceful plot lines."

Kilroy J. Oldster

I like to explain mindfulness not only by discussing the fact that you need to understand the triggers that cause certain emotions, but also through pointing out that we each have two different voices in our head. We have one voice which is self-aware and true to our best self, while there is another voice that lives in the moment and may offer false guidance by only looking to immediate satisfaction or desire. Kind of similar to the old and new mindset in Chapter Six. There's a constant battle between these voices, and it's up to you to make sure your self-aware voice wins.

How? By being more self-aware!

When you set a goal for yourself, this is your self-aware voice at work. This is you telling your own self that you want to do whatever it takes to achieve your goal. This is the voice that tells you, *I wish I could have her body* or *I wish I could be as athletic as him.* Then comes the other voice in your head, your living-in-the-moment voice, the voice that eventually steers you away from achieving your goal. The voice that tells you *Don't go to the gym today, stay at home* or *I'll eat this cake, as it won't do much harm.*

A common issue experienced by lots of people, including myself in the early stages of my journey, is that our living-in-the-moment voice almost always wins.

For some people, this voice is so strong and powerful that it causes them to drop out early in their journey. Others may be well into their journey, but because it can get overwhelming at times, their living-in-the-moment voice slowly takes over again and eventually sends them back to where they began—ground zero.

Again, I can't stress enough how important it is to realize that the journey is going to be a very bumpy ride. Not only in the early days, but throughout your journey, as well.

It's those who are mindless that relapse. It's those who are mindful that stay strong and overcome these mind-based challenges. Practicing mindfulness will not only help you distinguish between your self-aware voice and your living-in-the-moment voice, but it will also allow you to always make decisions based on your self-aware voice.

Decisions which are better and healthier for you.

Seriously. Always staying present and in control of your thoughts and emotions will take you closer and closer to reaching your goal, giving you a greater ability to sustain such a lifestyle.

The amount of times I experienced negative thoughts and emotions throughout my journey is countless. I can't stress to you enough how common this is for everyone looking to change their life—in any domain. Especially when it comes to transitioning into a healthy lifestyle, many different thoughts will be rushing through your mind.

On to this today, I experience those moments where my mind tells me not to go to the gym. Or those days where I feel like I want to eat anything and everything in front of me. This is all normal.

With time, I've learned to realize that this is just my *living-in-the-moment* voice talking—the voice I don't want to give any recognition to. When my mind tells me not to go to the gym, I kind of take a step back and understand why I don't want to go to the gym. I realize that it's not my body talking, because I feel good. It's just my living-in-the-moment voice providing false guidance. If I'm feeling fresh and physically ready, why not go to the gym? I understand it's this voice that's holding me back from achieving my goals, and so I don't want to give in. Instead, I go to the gym and end up feeling amazing afterward. It's only when you finish a workout session that you realize what a great decision you've made.

The feeling afterward is so rewarding.

To be mindful is to be present, and to be present is to be self-aware. By being self-aware, you'll *notice* and *know* the voices in your head. And when you know the voices in your head, you'll distinguish the self-aware voice from the *living-in-the-moment* voice. When you can differentiate between these two voices, you'll have the power to always listen to the self-aware voice.

This only comes through practice and consistency.

Again, it's going to be really hard. At first, you'll feel like your living-in-the-moment voice will always win.

But the more you're aware of these voices, and the more you practice listening to your self-aware voice, you'll end up having this voice as the driver of your thought process.

It's only when you have your self-aware voice in the driving seat that you'll realize yourself being immersed within a healthy lifestyle, easily and naturally. This is where I am now, and this is where I want you to be after reading this book.

Chapter 13
Emotional Eating

*"Don't let your mind bully your body into believing
it must carry the burden of its worries."*

Astrid Alauda

Emotional or stress eating means using food as comfort—not eating because you're actually hungry! Before I delve deeper into this area, you have to understand that there exist two types of hunger: physical and emotional hunger. The key is to know the difference between the two.

Emotional eating is when you eat because of emotions. You're not actually hungry. It's just you wanting to use food as a comfort to a problem you are having. Physical hunger is when you're hungry. It's not to the point of reaching starvation mode, to the point where you hear your stomach making weird noises and feel hunger pangs, but it is when you are hungry enough to eat your next main meal or snack. The key here is that you're not eating because you're just bored, anxious, sad, or stressed!

Emotional hunger is very powerful—because the mind is indeed really powerful.

However, it's only when you practice mindfulness that you can truly listen to your mind and body and then make healthier decisions. Mindful eating is about using physical cues to drive our hunger, not emotional cues related to comfort. There are some differences between the two, and it's important you know what they are to help you start practicing mindful eating.

Emotional Hunger	Physical Hunger
Happens suddenly	Happens gradually
Comes from the mind	Comes from the stomach
Leads to mindless eating	Leads to mindful eating
Craves comfort (unhealthy) foods	Craves healthy foods
Leads to regret and guilt	Leads to satisfaction and peace of mind
Doesn't make you full	Makes you full

Stress Eating

Emotional eating can be driven by a mix of emotions which lead to either under- or overeating. Stress eating, as the word describes, is more specifically related to the response of overeating due to stress.

So, why do we eat more when we are stressed?

First, stress increases cortisol levels. When cortisol levels are high, our craving for food increases. But unfortunately, it's not healthy foods that we seek out to satisfy these cravings. While the rise in cortisol increases cravings, it also increases hunger hormones, which makes us crave fatty and sugary foods. This is why stressed individuals always reach out for things like chocolate, chips, ice cream, or any other sugary or fatty food for that matter. It's why most of my clients who claim to live a stressful lifestyle are those who find themselves having so many cravings. While they think that their body needs it because they are simply *craving it*, what they're experiencing is actually the internal response in the body due to stress. In essence, and as I usually tell stressed eaters, cravings all start in the mind. Learn how to control your mind, and you'll learn how to control your stress eating.

A thousand years ago, life was very different from what it is today. We didn't have ticking clocks or imminent deadlines. There were no piles of paperwork, no internet, and no social media—there was less stress. Stress is dangerous, harming every aspect of your being. So, why not take back control and choose not to let it consume you? Whenever you feel overwhelmed, take a step back. Take a deep breath. Take a moment to reset, reboot, and recover. There are many ways to be mindful, even if it means just closing your eyes and thinking about the things that make you happy. Smile for a moment and remember why you're here.

Manage Your Emotions

Through practicing mindfulness comes learning to manage your emotions. When you manage your emotions, you'll find yourself better able to control your cravings and emotional/stress eating habits.

Different individuals experience various feelings. While some might feel stressed and eat more, others might feel stressed and lose their appetite. The same applies to feelings of boredom, depression, anxiety, frustration, and other negative emotions. Some may experience a huge appetite, and others no appetite whatsoever. Be aware of this, and pay attention to your own habits and triggers when it comes to stress and eating.

Here are ways you can practice mindfulness when finding yourself about to reach for the box of chocolates:

- **Take away temptations.** The simplest thing you can do is to just remove any unhealthy foods from your kitchen pantry or fridge. Don't even shop for such types of food, let alone keep them available in your kitchen. When you know you have these foods available, you'll subconsciously have the desire to reach out for them.

- **Find healthier alternatives.** Another simple strategy you can implement is to seek out healthier swaps. Buy dark chocolate instead of milk chocolate. Sweet potato chips or popcorn instead of regular chips. Protein bars instead of chocolate bars. Also, you can go to your local healthy bakery and buy healthier cookies, or chocolate bars which have raw and clean ingredients.

- **Drink water.** Rather than reaching for drinks like soda, or unhealthy food, drink more water. Sometimes hunger is due to a lack of fluid intake rather than a lack of food intake. Water may keep you more satiated and hydrated at a lower-calorie cost.

- **Talk to a friend or family member.** Sometimes during stressful times, we just need support. Rather than reaching for unhealthy comfort food, catch up with a friend or family member for a bit and perhaps even vent to them. You'll actually do yourself a favor by comforting yourself through talking to someone rather than eating comfort food.

- **Meditate.** Whether you want to just lay on the floor in silence and gather your thoughts, take deep breaths, or even use a meditation app, meditation is a great way to ease your mind and calm yourself.

- **Read.** Reading is an excellent way to distract yourself from negative thoughts and emotions. Take a break and read a chapter of a book or a magazine.

- **Exercise.** If you haven't exercised during the day, this could be an excellent opportunity to release stress and negative emotions. Move.

- **Practice yoga**. This is one of the best ways to combine exercise and mediation in one. Yoga is an activity I love and highly recommend you get into. It's a great way to strengthen the mind and body, and an even better way to calm your thoughts and emotions.

- **Take a walk.** I love doing this. It's not my go-to strategy, but it's definitely something I've done many times. When you take a walk alone, even if it's for ten minutes, you'll realize how much more at peace you'll feel with yourself. If you have a dog, perhaps take the dog with you. You'll still accomplish the purpose of solitary reflection here. You're stress levels or emotions will dip, and you'll walk back into your house by walking straight past the comfort foods and saving yourself the extra calories and sugar!

- **Play a game.** I don't like to incorporate much technology when it comes to finding ways to de-stress the mind, but if it means distracting yourself to avoid munching on unhealthy foods, then by all means use this tactic. Play a game on your phone or computer. If you have kids, perhaps play a game with them.

- **Listen to music.** Another favorite of mine, and something I do quite regularly. Listening to music and even downloading new music and creating new play lists on *iTunes* is

a fun and easy way to distract yourself from food.
If you're like me and do a lot of daydreaming when listening
to music, it can certainly ease your mind.

- **Keep a food diary.** If you find yourself in an emotional
  situation and end up eating mindlessly, write down what and
  how much you ate, how you were feeling at the time you ate,
  and whether you were actually emotionally or physically
  hungry (hunger check). Through keeping a food diary,
  you'll end up finding an underlying theme to what causes
  you to eat out of emotions. You'll start to understand
  the triggers, your emotions, and the food responses.
  With time, you will start being more of aware of these
  triggers, and find ways (like the strategies above) to solve
  them. This then leads to healthier eating, better food
  decisions, and an overall healthier you.

I know you might be reading this and thinking to
yourself, *There's no way I can do any of this. I can just take
the easy way out and eat food to comfort myself.* The thing is,
emotional eating can lead to unwanted eating, and this sort
of eating will be detrimental to your health and fitness goals.
If you truly want to lose weight, or achieve any other goal
you set for yourself, you need to do whatever it takes to
avoid activities such as emotional eating. Remember, if you
invest in yourself to develop a growth mindset, the emotional
eating will slowly disappear.

By engaging in one of these strategies, or maybe even finding a positive strategy that works best for you which I haven't
listed above, you'll learn how to comfort yourself through
ways other than food. Doing so will help you avoid weight
and fat gain, and accelerate you towards your goals.

Chapter 14
A Mindful Mind

"The best way to capture moments is to pay attention. This is how we cultivate mindfulness. Mindfulness means being awake. It means knowing what you are doing."

Jon Kabat-Zinn

After reading the last chapter, by now you should be aware of the difference between emotional and physical hunger. You should also know that emotional and stress eating stem from the mind, and that this is something which can be resolved. Again, you just have to practice mindfulness and dig deeper into your soul to find a solution. Through such practice, you can start to develop mindful eating habits.

I want to lay down one simple fact: Mindful eating is healthy eating. This is something I've learned over time, but also something from which I've seen clear results after practicing it, and after some clients have practiced it, as well. Mindful eating takes time, but changing this one simple element in your relationship with food and how you eat will do wonders for your health and well-being.

Believe me.

Mindful eating is all about being aware of your food, from the first step of buying food (grocery shopping) all the way through to eating your food. Although mindful eating is applied mainly to healthy food, it can actually be practiced when eating unhealthy food, too.

While I believe mindful eating encompasses different aspects of our relationship with food, since this book is all about filling your mind, let's start with that.

Think of Food Like You Do Being In A Relationship

Your relationship with food... this is the first thing you need to be aware of. Think of your relationship with food in the same way you consider being in a relationship with a significant other. Do you want to be with someone who only brings negativity to your life? Someone who doesn't care for you or want the best for you? I doubt your answer is yes. What about being in a relationship with someone who supports you and helps you grow? Someone who shines a positive light onto your life? Now, that sounds more like it.

This is the same way you should view food. You know that eating unhealthy food can be harmful to your health if engaged in over and over again. But what you don't know is how your quality of life can significantly improve if you sprinkle your diet with clean, whole, and unprocessed foods. On the inside, you'll feel clean, light, and healthy. You'll also have more energy throughout the day and experience better moods. On the outside, you'll attain the body you've always wanted. If you train daily, you're only enhancing your performance and recovery by choosing to eat the right foods. By doing so, you'll accelerate towards your body goals all the faster.

Choosing to eat healthy foods doesn't only impact your physical capacity; it affects your mental capacity, as well. Your brainpower and ability to think clearly will improve. Whether you work or study at school/university, your focus and concentration will massively improve. Eating clean and staying hydrated also improves mental performance during exercise. You'll make better decisions (this applies to non-exercise related daily activities, too), experience a quicker reaction time, and increase your fatigue threshold—this being the point at which you begin to feel fatigue and experience a decrease in exercise performance.

Another point to think of is knowing where your food came from, just like you want to know the person you're getting into a relationship with. You want to date or marry someone who you truly know and are certain of spending the rest of your life with! It's exactly the same principal with food. If you go grocery shopping, or just before you pick out what to eat, know more about the food you're about to eat. Where does it come from? How was it made? Was it grown? Is it processed or unprocessed? By doing this, not only will you strengthen your relationship with food, but you'll find yourself building better eating habits.

Improving your relationship with food doesn't stop there. Here are other ways to improve your relationship with food:

- **Focus on eating better.** Don't strive for perfect eating. Focus on how you can improve your eating habits and behavior and food choices.

- **Don't put yourself down.** If you've had one too many cheat meals or snacked on unhealthy foods, don't beat yourself up! Slip-ups happen. The key is to learn from your mistakes, understand why you messed up with your food, and then pick yourself back up.

It's about bouncing back, not going backwards.

- **Have balance.** Some people have the mentality to go all-in and be extremely healthy, and others go through phases of going all-out and binge eating. But there is no need to go through extreme behaviors. By eating in a balanced way, you'll improve your relationship with food.

- **Food as nutrients.** Thinking of food as nutrients, and understanding foods as functions, will allow you to make better food choices. Knowing the benefits healthy foods can have on the mind and body will allow you to continue eating in a healthy manner.

- **Enjoy your food.** Eat foods you enjoy. This is the best way to keep things exciting for you.

- **Be social.** Being healthy doesn't mean locking yourself in your room to avoid eating out or ordering in with family and friends. Eating is a social activity, and by enjoying these moments and meals, you can also improve your relationship with food.

All this being said, having a better relationship with food is fundamental to eating healthy. When you view food as something that will nourish your mind and body, as fuel to perform the best you can, and as a means to feeling good, you'll change not only the way you eat, but what you eat.

You Are What You Digest And Absorb

Have you heard the statement *You are what you eat?* While I really value this statement, I like to instead think of it as *You are what you digest and absorb.*

Eat healthy foods, and you'll digest properly and absorb the right nutrients to keep your mind and body feeling strong, healthy, and nourished. Do the opposite, and you'll lack the nutrients to keep you in top shape, mentally and physically.

I realized how powerful this statement was when I started to feel the benefits of eating healthily. Incorporating more fruits and vegetables into my diet, eating lean-quality proteins, healthy fats, and good carbs, and staying hydrated, was truly a game changer. I began to eat more regularly throughout the day in order to control my hunger and appetite levels, but also as a means of fueling and refueling my body to make sure I kept my muscle fuel tank full to improve my exercise performance. Since I had several classes throughout the day when I first started on this journey, I'd put in the time to pack healthy snacks like nuts and fruits to keep me energized and focused.

It's unbelievable how much healthy eating can change your quality of life, from the way you feel on the inside to how you reveal yourself on the outside. It's true that what you put into your body is what you will get out of it.

Eating healthy and unprocessed food gives your body nutrients and the good calories it needs to perform at the best level, mentally and physically.

You know what I realized the problem with unhealthy eating is, though? Sometimes we just don't feel the negative impact it has on our body. We don't actually see what's going on internally—the digestion and absorption of foods, the sugar spikes, the fat storage, and the harm to certain organs. Because of this, we continue our normal eating habits and behaviors.

For some, this can lead to constant unhealthy eating. It's only when you look at yourself in the mirror, hop on the weight scale, or wear a pair of jeans you bought a few months ago that you realize something has gone wrong.

So, how can you get past unhealthy eating and better understand what healthy eating can actually do for you? You have to focus on the feeling of living healthy, and how you feel before and after you eat. Continue reading on!

It's All About The Feeling

Today, we're bombarded with information more than at any other time in history. Social media plays a big part in this. Especially when it comes to health and fitness, we have so many influencers in the field, all of whom showcase their amazing bodies on their accounts. While I appreciate people using this as a means to motivate and inspire people, it associates health with just looking good. From a nutrition point of view, it tends to make people think of things from a pure weight and fat loss perspective for the sake of looking good.

But what happened to the *feeling?*

Many people ask me how I stay motivated to eat healthily. My answer to them is simply: *the feeling.* Indeed, it really boils down to how I feel after eating healthy as the thing that most motivates me to continue living this way.

Trust me, I've been in so many situations in the past where I've decided to cheat and eat junk food. To this day, I some-times do that (but to a much lesser extent). But time and time again, I've realized how horrible I feel afterwards. It's just not fun when I'm constantly bloated and experiencing irregular bowel movements. I start to guilt-trip myself and regret why I ate such foods, and so I only bring in more mental stress. I don't like this feeling at all!

Then I compare the way I feel when I eat healthy foods, and I just truly love the feeling. I don't suffer from bloating, cramps, or that gassy feeling in my stomach. I always feel light and clean afterwards, too. With all this comes feelings of awesomeness because I know that what I put into my body is beneficial, but also because I just feel good.

When I compare how I feel, both physically and mentally, after eating healthy vs. unhealthy foods, the way I feel after eating healthy foods is just unbelievable. As soon as I was mindful to these feelings, I asked myself, *Why the heck should I eat foods that will make me feel physically and mentally uncomfortable when I can make conscious decisions for eating and living healthily and simply feel amazing?*

I told myself, *I want to keep feeling this way!* And from then on, that's what I decided to do. Eat and live well to constantly feel amazing and energized.

It's all about the feeling, honestly. This is something I really want you to focus on, and to do so, you have to be mindful not only of what you eat, but how you feel before and after— and also your general feelings throughout the day. Once you're aware of the feeling and genuinely see the difference, believe me, you're going to love it and want to continue eating and living healthily for as long as you live. Here are some feelings to start paying attention to:

- Energy levels during the day

- Mood

- Focus

- Gut health – do you feel lighter? Less bloated?

- Exercise performance

- Work/studying performance (i.e. thinking clearer, having more concentration/focus, better decision-making)

- Sleep quality

You are what you eat or *You are what you digest and absorb:* Whichever statement resonates with you more, I really think you should take it seriously.

It's only when you understand that the food you eat can massively impact your body's internal mechanism that you will start to change the way you eat. The point is, food doesn't only impact the way you look or your exercise performance. It can hugely affect the way you feel on the inside. What determines the way you feel is what you digest and absorb, and what determines this is what you eat. Eat clean and healthily, and you'll do your body wonders and allow it to perform at its best by providing it with the right ingredients to keep you feeling strong and healthy. Even though you might not see what's going on internally, you'll most definitely feel it with time.

Let's face it, with all the research being done and the thousands of articles on *Google*, we all know that unhealthy eating does lead to unwanted health conditions.

So, why do it in the first place?

Think Before You Eat

Part of mindful eating is increasing your food awareness. Before you eat, you need to stop for a moment and think of what exactly you're putting into your body. I just mentioned to you that, while you may not feel like eating unhealthy foods is detrimental to your health, it certainly can cause negative side effects.

At the instance of eating, you won't feel the effects, and so, you'll continue to do it because you don't feel anything negative. Not to scare you or anything, but in the long-term, you'll most certainly feel these effects.

By practicing mindfulness, not only will you understand the negative internal bodily reactions, but you'll be more aware of the foods you eat. Mindfulness, in this sense, means always reaching for the cleaner food option and always ordering the healthier meal at a restaurant. When you're mindful, you'll increase your food awareness through knowing that choosing the healthy option will only benefit you. It's only once you experience these benefits that you'll continue to be aware.

Think After You Eat

Let's say you've had a long and stressful day at work, and you're dreading the idea of going back home to cook. So, you decide to stop by a fast food joint and pick up a quick and cheap meal. Do you ever notice how you feel right after the meal, or perhaps the next day?

Let me give you another situation in the same scenario. Instead of driving by a fast food restaurant and taking the easy but unhealthy route, you decide to go back home and dedicate forty-five minutes to roasting a chicken breast and some vegetables in the oven. How do you feel after the meal, or perhaps the day after?

Some food for thought, definitely.

I'm 100% sure you've felt much better physically after eating the home-cooked meal as opposed to eating fast food. You didn't get that *nasty* or *disgusting* feeling, nor the gas or bloating you would get after eating a greasy meal like you'd find from a fast food option. You most definitely did not experience the indigestion you would get after eating fast food!

Aside from the physical feeling, how do you feel mentally after eating a fast food meal vs. eating a healthy, home-cooked meal? Let me tell you that, more often than not, what you'll be thinking is, *Ugh, why did I eat that? I feel disgusting.* Yes, it may have been a delicious meal, but mentally, you're inviting feelings of remorse and guilt.

On the flip side, after eating a healthy meal, I'm sure you will feel awesome. Not only will you feel great physically, but also the fact that you ate a healthy meal makes you feel happy and proud of yourself that you've chosen the healthy route. Mentally, you'll be relaxed, too.

My point is, you need to be mindful not only *before* you eat, but *after* you eat, as well. Why put yourself through the physical and mental stress of eating unhealthily when you can just choose to eat right and invite in the positive feelings associated with being healthy?

It's a simple decision, but it's a decision YOU have to make.

Chapter 15
Mindful Eating

"Everything is created twice, first in the mind and then in reality."

Robin Sharma

Have you ever found yourself in a situation where you were working in the office or at home with a bag of chips or some chocolate on your desk, and when you looked down, *it had suddenly disappeared?* You'd been so focused on whatever task was at hand, you got to the point of finishing whatever it was you were eating without even noticing.

Yeah, that's *mindless eating* for you right there!

I'd be lying if I said I'd never been in that situation. It's a lousy feeling when you realize your food is gone and you've eaten so much without even thinking about it.

But this is exactly what happens when you're not mindful when you eat.

There are many ways to eat mindfully. It's also really important to know that mindful eating isn't an all-or-nothing approach.

You don't have to practice every point to be a mindful eater. Sure, it would be great if you could, but implement the strategies that work best for you and your lifestyle. Just like I'd say you should choose exercises that you enjoy to keep you committed for the long-term, choose mindful eating strategies that will actually help you to continue eating mindfully.

Here are some elements to consider:

Grocery Shopping

I mentioned previously that mindful eating starts with buying your food. It starts at the grocery store. I'm always aware of which aisles in the supermarket I should and should not be visiting. By being attentive and mindful, you'll be sure not to enter the aisles that tempt you to buy foods that you should otherwise not be eating!

Fill your cart with whole, clean, and unprocessed foods. Visit the fruit and vegetable aisles. If there's a healthy or organic section, go there, as well. It's best to always avoid the aisles where most of the candies, chocolates, chips, sodas, and canned juices are, just to avoid the temptation. On a side note, don't go grocery shopping when you're hungry. This was a trap I used to fall into, and it led to me filling the cart with the wrong foods!

Eat With an Appetite And Not When Starving

If you come to the table when you're starving, chances are that you're going to eat everything and anything in front of you, and in large portions, too. It's really important to start eating your meal when you're hungry, but not to the point of being starving. Of course, the feeling of starvation may be due to a really busy working day, coupled with a roller coaster of emotions that may reduce your appetite. In order to avoid that, it is best to eat every 3-4 hours throughout the day and drink 1-2 glasses of water every 1-2 hours. Thirst often masquerades as hunger when you are under-hydrated.

Control Your Portions

You know when I mentioned finding something that works best for you? This piece of the puzzle was the first thing I started with, and definitely the most effective for me. When I started to control my portions, not only did it change my physical appearance, it also made me realize how much food I was eating in unnecessary quantities. As humans, I think our evolution has worsened when it comes to health/nutrition, and some studies actually show this. We tend to move less and eat more. Our portions have increased significantly over the past 50 years or so, and this had led to the rise in obesity we're seeing around the world.

Here are some ways I've better controlled my portions:

Using The Hands

I don't believe in calorie counting, and nor do I believe in taking a scale with you wherever you go to measure how much you're eating. It's a waste of time and I don't believe it's a sustainable lifestyle. Instead, aim for using your hands as a reference for controlling your portions. Your hands are an amazing reference to use when it comes to portions.

First, your hands are with you wherever you go. Second, your hand size is generally representative of your body size and how much food you actually need. Note that for all serving sizes using the hands, recommendations are made on a per-meal basis (not the whole day) and may change depending on your goals and body size. This just serves as a general rule of thumb, no pun intended.

Protein

One serving size of proteins—such as chicken, beef, fish, eggs, or plant-based sources such as lentils, chickpeas, beans, and tofu—should be the size of your palm. Men should aim to eat two serving sizes (or 2x the size of their palm) at each meal. Women should aim for one serving size.

Carbohydrates

Carbohydrates such as rice, pasta, bread, and wholegrains should be equivalent to the size of your cupped hands. Again, men should consume 2x the size of their cupped hands, and women 1x per meal.

Healthy Fats

Healthy fats such as nuts, oils, avocado, and peanut butter should be the size of your thumb. Men should eat 2x the size of their thumb at each meal, and women one times.

Vegetables

Vegetables, including salads, should be the size of your clenched fist. While you may think salads and vegetables are healthy, so you can eat as much as you want, it is still useful to practice portion control even with such foods as these. As usual, men should aim to eat 2x the serving size and women 1x the serving size per meal.

1/3 Rule

Simply put, I'd portion my plate to 1/3 protein, 1/3 salad/vegetables, and 1/3 carbohydrates.

½ Rule

If for some reason I wasn't eating carbs in a given meal, I'd divide my plate into halves – ½ salad/vegetables and ½ protein.

Eat Slowly

When eating, especially if you're extremely hungry, it can be easy to eat fast to satisfy your hunger as quickly as possible. This is not the best practice. It's really important to take your time and to eat slowly. It takes twenty minutes for the brain to realize you're full. By eating slowly, you're actually doing yourself more of a favor because the slower you eat, the quicker your brain will tell you that you are full. Meaning, you'll stop eating, which usually equals out to consuming less food.

Chew More

Remember the term I used to refer to my early days of starting my health journey, *being sick in the head*?

This was one of the ways that defined me as being just that. I remember reading somewhere that you should count to thirty while chewing your food, to ensure that you break down the food properly to aid with digestion and ease your gut. Literally, I used to do that. It was pretty annoying, to be honest, but like I said, when it comes to being healthy you need to have that sort of obsessive behavior—at least in the beginning. Eventually, I got used to chewing more and dropped the whole counting thing.

With that being said, though, focus on chewing your food! If you think you can use the strategy of counting the number of times you chew, then aim for chewing 30-40 times before swallowing. Otherwise, just aim to chew more.

Take Small Bites

I found myself doing this a lot in the past, and still find myself doing this now. I've definitely learned to take smaller bites, whether using a spoon, fork, or biting from a sandwich. When you take smaller bites, not only will you taste your food more, but you'll also be able to chew more. It's a double whammy!

Don't Stuff Yourself

I always tell my clients to walk away from the table once they feel satisfied. My advice is the same to you. When you learn to notice the feeling of satisfaction and are able to walk away from the table or stop eating, you'll take one more leap toward your physical goals. It will make you realize how much extra and unnecessary food you are eating, and how much food you actually need.

This is a tough one because, when you're used to eating the amount you've become accustomed to versus what you actually should be eating, you may not necessarily feel full. When you start to practice this form of mindful eating, you may very well feel hungry at the point at which you think you are satisfied. Some people may give into this hunger and eat more, but others can stop more easily. I advise you to do your best to stop, and perhaps have a healthy snack a couple of hours after. Not only does this help you practice mindful eating, but with time, your stomach will actually adapt to the smaller quantities and you'll feel fuller more easily, and much faster than before. Eating regularly, too, as I've already alluded to, may help keep your hunger, appetite, and food cravings in check.

So, Why Should I Eat Mindfully?

You may be reading all this and thinking to yourself, *Why should I eat mindfully?* As you've noticed now, though, when you eat mindfully, you eat healthily. You're more aware of choosing the right foods and making better decisions. By understanding your physical and mental experiences, you can be more aware of the effects that food has on you, leading you to choose healthier foods. When you practice portion control, eat slowly, chew more, and take smaller bites, you'll find yourself feeling much lighter, and digesting and absorbing foods more efficiently.

Other than the food aspect, however, the ability to take control of yourself, emotions, thoughts, and decisions, and doing so comfortably and confidently, is a beautiful feeling. To lead your own path and have the ability to do things on your own without getting professional help is a great asset that you can use for the rest of your life.

Pillar 4: Sacrifice

Fill Your Mind Before You Fill Your Plate

Chapter 16
Organize Your Day
Around the Gym

*"Sacrifice is a part of life. It's supposed to be.
It's not something to regret.
It's something to aspire to."*

Mitch Albom

Without pain, there would be no suffering. Without suffering, we would never learn from our mistakes. To make things right, pain and suffering are the key to all windows, and without them, there is no way of bettering our lives. So, how far are you willing to go to be a healthier you? Are you willing to endure some pain in order to achieve your goals?

Will you sacrifice some comfort in order to become a healthier version of yourself?

Here's the answer: You must! It's part and parcel of living a healthy lifestyle, just like the rest of the pillars.

Taking you back to my university days, the *sick in the head days,* I can't tell you how much sacrificing I did in order to become the person I am today.

You've got to do it, and in so many different ways—nutritionally, physically, socially... the whole nine yards.

How far are you willing to go to achieve your goals? How much are you willing to sacrifice? Nothing will fall into your lap if you're not willing to work for it. We need to push harder, reach higher, and put our limits to the ultimate test. Sacrifice is the key to success in every aspect of your life. Rise earlier in the morning, and get a kickstart on your work. Resist temptations. Say no to unhealthy choices. Do one more push-up. Jog one more block. Prove to yourself that YOU hold the power and YOU are in control.

Whereas a lot of people organize the gym around their day, I used to organize my day around the gym. Of course, I used to prioritize my studies and other very important errands, but I would also fore go a lot of other things just so that I could hit the gym. During my university days, I'd go on trips to see friends, whether for a quick road trip to Virginia or flying across the country to the West Coast, and still make time to hit the gym. Even though I hadn't seen my friends for some time, I'd always have to sacrifice a bit of *chilling* time to go and hit the gym—even if it was for a 45-minute session. The fact that I did something and kept working out and staying in the routine comforted me more than anything.

If I was sick (not to the point where I couldn't move), I'd convince myself to go to the gym by thinking it would make me feel better. Obviously, I was living in denial. Sometimes, it wouldn't make me feel better and I'd pay the price, but even that never bothered me because going to the gym was what used to comfort me the most. The fact that I'd completed a very crucial daily task was the most important thing, and it made me feel accomplished for the day. So, yes, I did sacrifice my health sometimes, and in hindsight, this is probably not a best practice or good advice for you to heed, but it's part of the game—you have to figure out what works for you, and what you can sacrifice.

One of my other role models, Kobe Bryant, an ex-*Los Angeles Lakers* basketball player and, for me, the best athlete to ever play the game, once played through a really bad fever. And in the 2009-2010 season, he fractured his ring finger close to the tip, and yet still managed to lead his team to his fifth championship AND win the NBA finals as the MVP. Now, that's what I call sacrifice.

If I'm anticipating a busy week or a busy day, I sacrifice some sleep time and set my alarm to 1.5 hours before I'd initially have set my alarm, just to make time for the gym and be able to exercise. I did this as a student, and I still do this today. Rather than finishing up all of my work and errands and THEN hitting the gym, with a potential risk of missing my workout due to being too tired from working and running errands, I set my alarm earlier to get in a morning session. Internally, this makes me so much more relaxed and comfortable because I later know that I've gotten the workout out of the way and I can then go about my day with peace of mind on that front.

Starting the day by exercising also offers a great feeling. Don't get me wrong, I used to do the opposite some-times, thinking I'd have the willpower to hit the gym after I'd completed everything I needed to do... and then I'd end up missing the session. I'm sure this has happened to you, too.

For me, falling into this trap did two things: 1) it made me realize that I'm not prioritizing the gym by keeping it at the bottom of my list, and 2) it made me feel absolutely horrible and guilty for missing my workout session for the day.

So, by waking up earlier and sacrificing some sleep time, I'm able to prioritize the gym and avoid any feelings of remorse or guilt; in fact, I instead start the day with great energy, focus, and calmness.

With that said, though, there are many times where I'd wake up and tell myself, *Ahh, I just want to go back to sleep. I can't see myself training in the gym right now. Let me just go to the gym tomorrow....* But it's part of the challenge. Especially the mental challenge. It's part of the obstacles that I mentioned to you before, and which you need to overcome if you really want to see change. Because, if you keep getting defeated by the obstacles, you won't get anywhere.

If I kept shutting my alarm off, I wouldn't have gotten to the gym, and if I didn't get to the gym, I wouldn't have reached my goal. And if I didn't get to my goal, I'd get annoyed with myself. And that's a feeling I never wanted.

Chapter 17
Endure The Pain

"A hero is an ordinary individual who finds the strength to persevere and endure in spite of overwhelming obstacles."

Christopher Reeve

Sacrifice also comes through enduring pain to achieve your training goals. If you want to become more athletic, fit, or lean, or achieve any other body goal you have in mind, you have to train intensely (but smartly). You have to keep progressing and pushing yourself to continue seeing gains and improvements. This is key, and it's actually one of the principals of exercise. To see changes in muscle, you need to overload your muscles and progress through different training methods and techniques. Overload and progression come with pain, believe me. As they say, *No pain, no gain. I* hate using cliché statements, but it's so true.

There have been other times where I've found myself working out through soreness—again, to let not go of the habit of skipping workout days. Honestly, the gym used to make me feel better. It was tough at first, getting my sore body to the gym, let alone getting it to work out, but by just being active and stimulating blood flow, the soreness I felt was actually reduced. But again, I exercised through the soreness and the pain that came with it, and that's my whole point. You have to endure some pain and fight through it to achieve your goals.

Nutrition Sacrifice

In the beginning of your healthy lifestyle journey, you may find yourself letting go of some (not all) of the foods you like. Sacrificing such things can be easier when you realize your purpose—WHY exactly you're putting yourself through any situation. Nutritionally, I knew that it would play a huge part in the person I wanted to be, and the person I wanted to look like. So, I just had to do it. I really believed in my goal and in my vision, and I wanted to do whatever it took to reach that goal. That's sacrifice.

Sacrifice is a test of how badly you really want something.

You have to resist temptations and sacrifice the *good stuff*—the desserts, chocolates, and all that. To be very honest with you, I was fortunate enough to go cold turkey and have it work in my favor. I don't recommend that you go cold turkey when cutting out any food temptations, but it did work for me. That said, I was never one to have a huge sweet tooth. Though it was very tough to cut out sweets and candy, I found other ways to deal with those cravings and overcome the mental temptations.

Let me give you an example.

If at times I used to crave something sweet after lunch or dinner, instead of reaching for a chocolate bar, I'd chew 3-4 pieces of a sugar-free, flavored gum to compensate for the sweet taste. As ridiculous as this may sound, it's the truth, and it worked! This goes to show you my obsession once again.

Most of the time, though, I'd just resist the temptations. It was a decision I used to make and a decision that worked the best for me. With time, I actually came to realize that my cravings and temptations lessened, and now I find myself not having many temptations to begin with, let alone giving in to them. All because I sacrificed in the beginning and went through some pain (more mental pain, in the case of temptations).

It may not necessarily be your sweet tooth that you find yourself sacrificing, but instead, foods like bread and pasta. Honestly, in my opinion, these foods do not necessarily have to be sacrificed. What you may have to sacrifice is the amount you eat (this is very relative, depending on your goals). If you've had 1-2 pieces of bread, is there a need to reach for a third piece? Or maybe you need to take smaller portions? This is where resisting temptations comes into play.

Social Sacrifice

Throughout your healthy lifestyle journey, social events are undoubtedly among the obstacles you will experience. Whether you are invited for lunch to your family's house or going out to dinner with you friends on a Friday night, you will probably feel the need to sacrifice just a bit. Let me tell you how I did it.

There were a few things I did, or gave up, to make sure I was staying on the right track. First, if I was going out to eat with friends, I'd do one of two things: 1) prepare and eat a home-cooked meal beforehand so that I didn't mess up at that meal, or 2) I would go out with my friends and resist the temptation of ordering an unhealthy option on the menu by eating something healthier. Remember how I mentioned checking out a restaurant's menu ahead of time and planning in advance?

That's key in a case like this!

In both cases, there was something I had to let go of. In the first scenario, I'd sacrifice a potentially delicious (yet somewhat unhealthy) meal at the restaurant by not eating with my friends. In the second scenario, I'd sacrifice only the particular meal. In both cases, though, I was out with my friends—which, to me, is also important. At the time of my *sick in the head* phase, eating what they ate was not important! I have gotten called out on this and teased, but in my mind, I always knew I had the last laugh because I was making the right decision of eating a healthy meal and doing my health a favor.

This is an important point I want you to really under-stand—that if you want to live a healthy lifestyle, you have to let go of certain things in order to really see change and results. Additionally, you have to withstand some of the peer pressure and embarrassment that comes with eating healthy. But what should keep you strong and happy through this process is the fact that it should NOT be embarrassing to eat healthy. You should not be getting teased if you are eating healthy. And so what if you are? You are doing absolutely the right thing by either eating before going out or eating healthy foods while sitting at the same table as your friends.

There's no shame in that!

Chapter 18
Exercise Your Willpower

"Don't let mental blocks control you. Set yourself free. Confront your fear and turn the mental blocks into building blocks."

Dr. Rooplen

We need to 'ex'ercise. However, we need to 'in'ercise, too. During my transition into a healthy lifestyle, as you now already know, there were some things I let go of and some feelings I had to fight. This is all part and parcel of trying to be a healthier you. As I keep saying, nothing involving change is smooth sailing.

One thing that I did during my journey was exercising my willpower.

Think about this for a second. If you want to get bigger and stronger, you have to exercise your muscles. The more you exercise, the more your muscles will adapt and start responding to the stimulus of promoting muscle growth or strength. If you stop exercising, your muscles start to lose size and strength. This is the exact same concept as exercising your willpower. The more you exercise or practice it, the stronger it will get, and the stronger YOU will get. The less you exercise it, the less willpower you have, and the more cravings and temptations you'll give into.

Take it from me. Throughout my journey, I had to hold myself back many times. I knew that if I did, though, I'd get better and better at resisting whatever the temptation was and eventually make it easier to curb my cravings. From resisting desserts to trying as much as I could to eat healthy whenever I was out with friends or family, I kept on exercising my willpower to make sure I always stayed in touch with my goals.

Here is my advice on ways to exercise your willpower:

- **Challenge yourself.** Take up a challenge or do something that you don't really want to do. Whenever you feel like you want to give up, don't! Stick with it and keep doing the task you set for yourself.

- **Don't overdo it.** When exercising your willpower, don't do too many things at once to try and test yourself. Focus on one thing at a time, or else you really will exhaust yourself and go back to square one.

- **Talk to yourself.** This isn't as weird as it sounds! It's just setting up a promise to yourself. For example, if I anticipated a sugar craving later in the day, I used to tell myself: *If I get a sugar craving, I'll eat fruits* or *If I'm craving a chocolate bar, I'll eat a protein bar instead.* When you talk to yourself and make such promises, consciously, you'll make it much easier to exercise your willpower.

Believe me, once you continually practice your willpower, you'll find it much easier to resist temptations, curb cravings, and make healthier decisions. Everything comes with time, patience, and consistency. Today, I find myself not having nearly so many temptations and cravings as I used to. When people hear me say this, they think I'm either joking or one of those people who deprives themselves the joy of eating food. Honestly, though, I genuinely mean it. I can easily say no to a piece of cake or dessert if it's put out in front of me now. Easily. The point is, though, that wasn't always the case—it came from practicing my willpower.

The best part of exercising your willpower and really having the strength to stick with things is that, when the time comes where you actually do give in to something, you won't fall into a cycle after that. For example, if I have a *cheat meal* one day, eating what I know I shouldn't, I can rest assured because I know I have strong willpower, and that I can wake up the next day and start on a fresh note and be healthy again, comfortably—and without going back to square one. I don't have any feelings of guilt or remorse, and I won't continue the cycle of unhealthy/cheating behavior. So, this is one huge benefit of exercising your willpower.

Yes, it's very tough and it does take time, but when you reach the point where you have a strong enough willpower to make a healthy lifestyle a part of you and your routine, everything will be second nature. Even if you mess up with your food, or skip gym days here and there, you'll have the confidence and ability to get back to your normal ways— your healthy ways.

Pillar 5: Habits

Chapter 19
Fill Your Mind

"Change might not be fast and it isn't always easy.
But with time and effort, almost any habit
can be reshaped."

Charles Duhigg

When I came up with these pillars, I strategically placed *Habits* as the last one. Not because it's the least important, but because of the fact that it's hard to make something a habit when you don't precede it with the right foundation. That foundation is the four pillars before it. Changing a habit is a very difficult and long process. It becomes an easier and more pleasant one when you develop a strong mindset, believe in yourself, live mindfully, and prepare to make sacrifices.

A habit is something which is so engrained in your brain that you perform it without thinking. Developing habits allows your brain to work on autopilot. In a way, our brain is lazy; it just takes thoughts, emotions, and behaviors and automates them.

In other words, your brain forms habits for you.

So, how are habits formed and what are their characteristics? Neuroscientists have found that habits have common features:

- They are triggered by something (a cue, situation, or event).
- They are learned over time due to constant repetition.
- They are formed automatically and with not much awareness.
- They are hard to break.

Neuroplasticity

Before delving deeper into habits and behaviors, you need to understand a bit of neuroscience, especially in relation to neuroplasticity. Again, I don't want to get too technical on you, but this will help you understand why it's sometimes so hard to break habits.

According to the medical definition of neuroplasticity, it is the *brain's ability to reorganize itself by reforming new neural connections throughout life.*

Speaking in the most basic language, a habit is made up of neural connections which are typically formed over a long period of time. Think of washing your hands every time you use the toilet, brushing your teeth before bed, or even flossing your teeth after every meal. What happens is that, through these actions, you wire your brain in a certain way that eventually makes such actions second nature. As with the examples above, sometimes you don't even realize that you're doing them because of how used to them you are! As you repeat something over and over again (and this repetition can be just as simple as the things you tell yourself), you strengthen the connections between the neurons in the brain. Eventually, they wire together and form a habit. When you turn thoughts into habits, this is pretty much what neuroplasticity, or brain plasticity, is all about.

The interesting thing here, which you may have already realized, is that our brains are plastic. Meaning, a brain can reorganize itself and wire thoughts differently. What does that mean? It means, YOU have the ability to rewire and reorganize your brain. It's only YOU who has the control to break bad habits and develop new and positive ones. As you now know, yes, it may take a lot of time, but it is certainly possible to achieve!

Chapter 20
Break Those Habits That Break You

*"A nail is driven out by another nail;
habit is overcome by habit."*

Erasmus

So, how do you break bad habits? In the previous chapter, I mentioned that habits are formed in several ways, and some of their characteristics are:

- Habits are triggered by a cue, situation, or event.

- Habits are hard to break.

We have to learn how to break the habits by:

- Understanding the trigger (cue, situation, or event).

- Wiring a new habit to break the old habit.

If you remember from the previous chapters, I talked about the old vs. the new mindset. In this chapter, I'll revisit that topic again, but this time in relation to habit change. When it comes to changing your habits, know that it's going to be quite uncomfortable to change habits and then maintain that change. This is not because your new habit is hard to adopt; it's simply because of the fact that your brain is wired to a specific pattern and routine. So, when you start to do things that will rewire your brain, it will feel uncomfortable and difficult, likely requiring a lot of time and effort.

Indeed, developing a new habit and replacing bad habits with more positive ones will take a lot of mental energy from you. You are essentially changing the way your brain works—replacing a wired and automatic habit with a new one. There will be so many moments where you will feel the need to fall back on your old habit because of feelings of ambivalence and discomfort. Any sort of change in life is scary and difficult, though, so don't worry about these hurdles because this is absolutely normal.

The key is not to completely avoid adopting the new habit when you feel this way, but to instead embrace it.

The third pillar of living a healthy lifestyle is *mindfulness.* When you're mindful, you can understand the thoughts and emotions that are running through your mind during a tough time—like when you're trying to undergo a habit change. Mindfulness can allow you to move past feelings of ambivalence and have the strength to fight negative feelings throughout the change process.

Being mindful can also allow you to pay attention to the trigger. And this is what is first needed in order to break a bad habit. You need to understand the trigger to make necessary changes. Once you do understand it, you need to mindfully and consciously repeat your new thought, behavior, or action to then start forming a new habit. If you've made your current (old) habits a habit, then by all means you can make your newly desired habit a habit, as well. Similar to how your old habit developed with time and repetition, your new habit needs to be formed in the same way—repeating the process many times over a long period.

Let me share with you my experience.

After moving into an apartment nearby UMD, I had one major problem, which was always craving something sweet after eating a meal, especially after lunch. I used to find myself browsing through the kitchen drawers, searching for anything sweet to change the taste of my mouth (the trigger).

This was an old habit, and now it's long gone. Why? Because I was fortunate enough to realize the trigger and do something else to divert my attention away from finding something sweet—I changed my habit.

So, after finishing lunch, instead of lingering around the kitchen, I'd resist the temptation and walk straight to my room in order to avoid the trigger and create a new response—all in order to stop having the temptation to eat something sweet. Eventually, with time and practice, I adopted this new habit (of resisting the temptation and avoiding the trigger), and now find myself rarely craving anything sweet after any meal. I was aware of the trigger and did something about it to start wiring a new habit in my brain.

For some, a trigger to eating unhealthy foods can be watching TV. Some people may not realize this trigger, and so they keep finding themselves munching on unhealthy snacks and, before they know it, they complain about putting on weight! It's only when the trigger is identified, in this case watching TV, that a new response can be formed.

Now, I'm not necessarily telling you to stop watching TV

all together. However, when you are aware of the fact that watching TV causes you to munch on unhealthy snacks, you may be mindful enough to either not munch at all, eat healthier snacks instead, or do something else other than watching TV to elicit a different response.

Going back to my example, I jumped straight to the conclusion of adopting a new habit, without mentioning anything in between. The old habit never seemed to die! It was always there, and there were so many times where I would want to give in, but had to tell myself to do otherwise. In fact, though, there were times where I relapsed.

When I started to make the transition toward a new habit, I recognized the cue that would cause me to eat sweets after lunch—the craving of something sweet itself. After lunch, I'd linger around the kitchen, opening the fridge and kitchen drawers to find anything sweet. I wasn't hungry—I just finished lunch—but I still wanted to eat something sweet!

This was the cue: the craving for something sweet after lunch. Now that I knew of the cue, I wanted to test it.

The first few occasions after this realization, rather than sticking around the kitchen, I would go straight to my room. No searching, no nothing. Going straight to my room rather than sticking around in the kitchen helped me avoid the temptation. The first few times were very difficult. The thought of wanting to go back to the kitchen and find something sweet was always on my mind. I really had to control myself in order to not go into the kitchen and rummage through the cupboard for something sweet. With time, however, I realized that my situation got better. Not only that, but my new habit of going straight to my room rather than sticking around in the kitchen eventually took over. I was able to rewire my brain and develop a better habit while letting go of an old habit.

This is not to say that I didn't experience moments of relapse. I definitely did. Nothing is easy and completely smooth sailing, as I've mentioned time and again throughout this book.

There were times when I would stick around the kitchen after a meal and find and eat something sweet. But I never beat myself up over it, and I most certainly did not let it cause a chain reaction of continually eating something sweet after the following meals. I enjoyed the moment, ate whatever it was I was craving, and carried on with my day... but I also made sure I didn't repeat this relapse again in the meals thereafter.

With that said, that's my first piece of advice to you when trying to replace bad habits: Don't put yourself down and definitely don't let any relapse cause a chain reaction.

Secondly, if you do want to replace an old habit—say, munching on unhealthy foods while watching TV or while on a business call, or in whatever situation it may be that you find yourself usually munching on food—then, 1) find a healthier alternative, and 2) be mindful of your portions. This is all a part of living a healthy lifestyle, which, like I said previously, includes mindful eating; in this sense, that means controlling your portions and increasing food awareness.

If you let loose, there's no need to let loose many times after that and then completely relapse with no plan of bouncing back. The key is to not repeat that same behavior and then make it a habit again. Pick yourself back up and embrace the moment while you can. Cut yourself some slack, and continue to focus on rewiring your brain for a new and better habit.

Break those habits that break you.

Chapter 21
Take It One Habit At A Time

"Your little choices become habits that affect the bigger decisions you make in life."

Elizabeth George

Throughout my health journey, I had so many goals in my mind. I wanted to do so many things—from hitting the gym to eating well, to trying to fix my sleep. I was telling you before that transitioning to a healthier lifestyle is not easy, and I certainly experienced that. Because of all the things I wanted to fix about myself, I ended up feeling stressed and frustrated on so many occasions. I just couldn't handle the responsibility of fixing everything all at once!

Being a student at the time, I couldn't really afford to pay a mentor or a health/lifestyle coach. So, I decided to do things on my own. This is where my love for self-help books developed. I started to dig into books and figure out strategies to better myself, especially looking for ways to improve habits and behaviors.

One common theme I came across was to focus on one habit at a time. This would allow me to put all of my attention and effort on one task at hand and try to nail it down as much as I could before moving on to anything else.

As hard as it was at first to focus on one habit only, especially since there were other things I wanted to improve, it really made a difference when I focused on one thing at a time. Before I pinpointed which habit it was that I wanted to focus on, I considered what should be my highest priority. Exercise. I just wanted to properly start working out on an everyday basis and get in the groove of being physically active. This was also the thing that would make me look as fit as those athletes I used to see around campus!

Exercise it was. This was what I was going to focus on until I saw both changes in the rewiring of my brain: the habit of going to the gym daily, and the confidence to move onto another habit, knowing that going to the gym had indeed become a habit of mine.

So, you may be wondering, how do I know if something is a habit?

Well, it's when you're confident enough that the new habit you are trying to form is truly something that will stay with you and which has become a part of who you are. On that note, my advice to you is the following: Prior to focusing on another habit, make sure that the current habit you are trying to form is one that is ingrained within you and feels like it is second nature to you. If you're not sure, think about whether it would feel unnatural to go without the habit for a few days. Would you miss it? Would you feel like your day was missing something? If not, it may very well be that it's not quite second nature yet and needs some more time in your focus.

The first few years of my transition, I was on a bulking phase at the gym. Not because it was intentional, but because I only wanted to focus on exercising without having to think about things like eating right. If you don't know it already, in order to gain weight or *bulk-up*, you need to be consuming more calories than you're burning. During this phase, sometimes it's a good idea to eat calorie-dense foods since you need more calories to grow bigger. That was my mindset at the time. While I didn't think of the food aspect due to effective habit-changes, I also didn't really care about what I ate. After all, it did help with my gym goal. So, this actually helped me with trying to focus on just the exercise part. To this day, my friends call me out on this time period. They tease me over how big I was (even though I didn't think I was as big as they made it seem).

It wasn't until 2013 that I was comfortable enough about the gym to focus on another habit. That's FIVE years! I've never really thought about this until now, actually, but it's true. It didn't necessarily take me five years to develop a habit, because you can develop a habit far faster than that if you just keep practicing and practicing, but I still can't believe it took me five years to transition into my next habit change focus. But that's exactly what I mean—habit change and change in general takes time!

At this point, I've gone through about five years of hitting the gym at least five times per week. It definitely became a habit of mine. I absolutely loved it once it got to be my habit, and I still hit the gym at the same frequency. Okay, maybe four times now because of yoga (either at home or in a studio), but that still counts as exercise! So, technically, I'm still exercising five times per week.

Going back to 2013, when I moved to the UK to take up my Master's degree, I was in the groove of exercising and it was time to move on to focusing on my next problem habit. Food. Not only was I confident enough to lose my focus on prioritizing the gym, because it had become second nature to me, but my exercise goals had changed. As a result, I had to change the way I ate. I was no longer bulking up. I wanted to start getting ripped and lean. Opposite to bulking up, in order to lose weight/fat and get more lean, you need to be burning more calories than you're consuming—so that's what I did. I started to eat less (but also with a focus on healthier food) while also exercising more. Because exercise was a habit of mine, it was easier to turn up the dial and exercise with more intensity to burn more.

Now it was time to focus on the food.

Today, I find myself having a completely different physique than I had five years ago. I'm definitely much smaller than before, but I am leaner. I think I can do better, and I actually want to since I haven't yet fully reached my goal, but I'm happier this way. The bulking phase was fun and all—eating whatever I wanted and not having to worry about all that—but I absolutely prefer my current look. I'm also a short guy, so being more lean suits me more than being short and bulky. I was able to be more lean due to already having adopted exercise as a habit, but also due to the simple fact that I was finally able to focus only on my food habits.

What I'm trying to get to with all this is that, if you want to change your lifestyle, if you want to change your habits, don't try to do everything at once. You're only going to cause more stress and frustration for yourself, and eventually you'll relapse and not go ahead with your plan.

Sit down with yourself and figure out the most important thing YOU want to do. I know you might have several priorities, but try to think of ONE that resonates with you the most right now. That one thing that you truly and deeply want to achieve.

When I work with my clients, I work with them in this way. I've worked with many who have more than one *bad* habit. For example, they drink soda on a daily basis while also having a big sweet tooth for chocolate. At the onset of our habit-change journey, I make the client decide which one they want to change first based on what their priority is, and also based on what they think is consuming their life the most. If it's the soda drinking, then we'll focus only on lessening their soda consumption while continuing to eat chocolate. It's only when the client demonstrates their ability to confidently reduce (if not completely replace their soda-drinking habit with, say, water) that we'll then move onto the next habit, chocolate.

If you were to start on your own without the guidance of a nutritionist, some examples to help with habit transformation that you may choose from are the following:

- Drinking water with every meal
- Eating five servings of fruit and/or vegetables per day
- Eating a source of protein at every main meal or snack
- Eating high-quality carbohydrates
- Cutting out all sugary drinks

Having said all this, don't try to exhaust yourself by doing too much all at once. You'll do yourself more harm than good. Take it slow, and as I mentioned in Chapter 7, take the baby step approach.

Take it one habit at a time.

Chapter 22
Believe Nutrition Habits

*"Find ways to learn that fit into your lifestyle
so you can adopt them as habits."*

Pascha Kelley

Working with clients, I focus on food as well as eating habits and behavior. Over the years, I have developed a habit-based curriculum whereby I incorporate certain habits to trigger behavior change within my practice. Let us delve deeper into some of these habits, which of course you can work on improving in your own life.

Eat Regularly

Changing bad habits gives you greater flexibility, which you can then harness in situations that test your willpower. Your first step on a journey of habit change and self-improvement is to eat regularly.

Planning healthy meals isn't difficult. Though, if you're not used to it, the planning can take a little practice. A healthy breakfast is a key start to the day. If you skip breakfast because you want to sleep a few minutes more, you skip out on essential nutrients and benefits that can improve your day. Include three meals and two snacks to keep you feeling satisfied all day long.

It's okay to make variations that fit your lifestyle and needs. Just do your best to incorporate healthy choices into your day—fruit, vegetables, lean proteins, beans, legumes, and whole grains are always smart bets.

Stop Sugar Cravings

Do you love the taste of something sweet? Do you constantly want more?

Even though we know sugar is not a nutrition choice, our body can frequently crave it. And, often, it can be hard to resist sugar cravings. We can crave sugar for several reasons, the main reasons being low blood sugar, high stress levels, and low energy.

Eating too much sugar (like sweets, fizzy drinks, and chocolate) creates a surge of feel-good brain chemicals called dopamine and serotonin.

Just like a drug, your body craves more after the initial high. You become addicted to that feeling, so every time you eat it, you want to eat more. Too much sugar raises your blood sugar, causing your pancreas to release insulin in an attempt to bring this level down. When more and more insulin is circulated in your blood stream, your body attempts to convert sugar into fat and stores it as an energy reserve. As a result, this can make you gain weight. The more sugar you eat, the more insulin is produced, which can lead to health problems such as insulin resistance and type-2 diabetes.

Feeling sluggish all the time or always being hungry or thirsty can all be signs you've been binging on too much sugar. Additionally, if you are only eating simple sugars, you will not get enough of the other nutrients (like protein and fiber) to sustain your energy.

Sugar cravings affect everyone. The key to dealing with them is knowing why you're getting them in the first place and making necessary changes to lessen them in the future. Having a healthy plan in place to deal with them in a conscious manner can also be a big help.

Do you need as much sugar as you think? Not really. Actually, something you can do is train your taste buds to enjoy foods that are not too sweet. Then, over time, begin to cut sugary foods out so that you don't feel the need to eat something sweet all the time. Here's what you can do:

- If you are having tea or coffee, slowly cut down on the additional sugar and syrups that are often added to such drinks. If you already drink black coffee, or tea without any sugar, then well done!

- Limit intake of sugary cereals, especially in the morning. Healthier alternatives such as oatmeal/porridge or whole wheat cereals are a better option.

- Cut out one sweet food from your nutrition plan each week.

- If you are the type to eat something sweet after main meals, perhaps reduce this indulgence; choose one meal a day when you'll avoid having something sweet after finishing your meal.

- Increase protein intake. High protein intake can make you feel full for longer and doesn't raise blood sugar levels like refined carbs and sugars.

- Increase fiber intake through fruits and vegetables.
  Like protein, fiber can make you full for longer, control your
  sugar cravings, and maintain your blood sugar levels.

- Drink more water.

- Choose healthier sweet options such as fruits, dried fruits,
  flavored yogurt (with no added sugar), dark chocolate,
  and protein bars.

- Exercise! Once you exercise, you'll start to change the way
  you eat. Aside from the benefits exercise can provide,
  by also eating better, you'll feel much better.

- Limit even healthy sugars like brown sugar and honey.
  Even though a food like honey may have benefits, it is still
  sugar at the end of the day.

Know Your Eating Triggers

What makes you eat?

Each of us has different eating triggers, and some might
be more obvious than others. Learning to recognize your
own eating triggers will help you figure out how to manage
them better. These are some of them:

- Certain places and actions may trigger you, like sitting down
  in front of the TV or watching videos on *YouTube/Snapchat/
  Instagram*

- Seeing and/or smelling food

- Emotions like stress or sadness

- Boredom

- Socializing with friends

- Exercise

By planning ahead and bringing awareness to trigger situations, you can successfully manage these weight-loss challenges.

Ten Minutes Per Day

Take ten minutes of alone time or stillness for yourself each day. It really does the trick for relaxing the mind. Whether you can sit in a quiet room with no technology for ten minutes or meditate for ten minutes, try as much as you can to have some down time.

Personally, I like to use meditation mobile applications as a way of getting this down time and as a way to practice meditating. I use *Headspace* and/or *Insight Timer*—check them out; they're really great!

Of course, the longer you can meditate every day, the better. But you have no idea how these few minutes of your day can impact your mind. Meditating for ten minutes on a daily basis (or as much as you can during the week) can really change the way you see the world and can also change your physical fitness.

Think of meditation as a window into your mind. The more you meditate, the more you clean this window, making it clearer and easier to see through. It's the same thing with meditation and the mind. Meditation will help you think more clearly and put you in a more balanced state of mind.

Say No!

Have you ever been in a situation where you felt shy or embarrassed about saying no to eating unhealthy foods in front of family and friends? If you have, then this habit is for you!

There is no shame in saying no to people if they offer you unhealthy foods. There is also nothing wrong with eating a healthy meal when your friend or family is eating an unhealthy meal right next to you. There is absolutely nothing wrong with that. If anything, you are becoming the role model by eating healthy.

To be honest, this habit might take some getting used to. It's tough to say no to family and friends, and it's also tough to say no to chocolate and fries. But believe me, once you get used to saying no, it will do you wonders and it will only help you achieve your goal faster.

Section 3

Nutrition for the Mind

Chapter 23
Sleep Hygiene

"True silence is the rest of the mind, and is to the spirit what sleep is to the body, nourishment and refreshment."

William Penn

Sleep is an often overlooked area when it comes to living a healthy lifestyle. The fact of the matter is, sleep can play a huge role in the way you eat.

First and foremost, we know proper sleep can have the same effect on the mind as healthy eating. By experiencing good sleep quality and a sufficient quantity of it, we can enhance focus and concentration, improve mood, increase energy levels, and make more health-conscious food decisions. But, sleep also improves your physical health, as well. For instance, we know that one of the best times, if not the best time for your body to recover from exercise and in general, is during sleep!

So, what is sleep hygiene? According to the *National Sleep Foundation,* sleep hygiene is *a variety of different practices and habits that are necessary to have good nighttime sleep quality and full daytime alertness.*

Basically, there are things you can do prior to sleeping which can really improve on the time it takes for you to fall and stay asleep, along with improving the overall quality of your sleep.

Here are some ways to improve sleep hygiene:

- **Sleep in a dark room.** You may already know this, but it's extremely important. The darker your room, the better you'll sleep. Of course, I know some people may need some sort of light in order to fall asleep. If anything, keep this at a minimum and perhaps avoid having the light source close to your bed—you don't want it to be a bedside lamp, for example.

- **Sleep in a quiet room.** If you live with friends, family, or have roommates, it's important to let them know when you plan to sleep so that they can (hopefully) keep the noise levels down. Sleeping in a noisy environment negatively affects the time it takes for you to fall and stay asleep. Shhh!

- **Set the temperature anywhere between 18-20 degrees Celsius.** Science shows that this is an ideal temperature to improve sleep quality. For some, this may be too cold. The point here is to make sure that you don't sleep in too cold or too hot of an environment.

- **Sleep and wake up at regular times.** Our body has an internal body clock and is highly affected by our sleeping patterns. The more you can wake up and sleep at regular times, the more stable and adjusted your body clock will be. In turn, this will keep your biological clock in check and allow your body functions to perform at optimal levels.

- **Avoid technology 30-60 minutes before bed.** All of the above points are important, but this one is especially important to pay attention to, given the era we live in.

Mobile phones, laptops, and tablets are highly utilized in today's age. The habit of using mobile phones or any other device prior to sleeping, as a way to fall asleep, may actually be the cause of sleep disruption. The fact of the matter is that the blue light from such devices actually disrupts sleep, negatively affecting both quantity and quality.

So, now that you know more about sleep hygiene, what are some things you can do to further help your sleep and improve mind and body power?

- **Limit caffeine intake before going to sleep.** Caffeine remains elevated in the blood for around 10 hours. Even if you are a big-time coffee or tea drinker and have a high tolerance for caffeine, it would still be best to avoid any caffeine source in the afternoon if you want to improve sleep quality and quantity.

- **Take a hot bath or shower.** It's true, taking a hot shower before sleeping can calm your mind and body, which will put you in a tranquil state before sleeping and thus help you sleep well.

- **Read.** Whether you read a book, magazine, or newspaper, reading before sleeping can take your mind off a busy working day you may have had or any other issue you may have at hand. Plus, you don't get any blue light from technological devices.

- **Drink herbal teas.** Chamomile, lavender, and valerian root are all ingredients you should look out for in herbal teas. These compounds can aid with relaxation prior to sleeping and are a much better alternative than caffeinated beverages.

- **Meditate.** Whether you have your own ritual, use a guided meditation app, or do something like focusing on your breathing, meditation is a fantastic way to help relax your mind and take your mind off of your daily stresses. Some mobile apps that I have used in the past to help with guided meditations include *Calm, Head Space,* and *Insight Timer.*

So, why mention sleep? And how does it relate to nutrition? Well, for starters, we know sleep plays a huge role with brain function. Good sleep can improve your decision-making and problem-solving abilities. It can increase energy, focus, and concentration, and even positively impact your mood.

All of this, in turn, can impact your food choices and nutrition. Science shows that there is indeed a correlation between sleep and nutrition. The better we sleep, the better food choices we make, and the healthier the foods we eat. The opposite happens when you lack good quality and quantity of sleep, which leads to choosing foods that are higher in calories, fat, and sugar. This, of course, may lead to weight gain.

When trying to living a healthy lifestyle, focus on your sleep just as much as you focus on anything else. You need proper sleep to focus on whatever task you have at hand anyway.

Sleep like a baby.

Chapter 24
Feed Your Brain

"Health is a relationship between you and your body."

Terri Guillemets

As a part of being mindful in your healthy lifestyle journey, I mentioned that it is important to focus on the feeling rather than looks only. Part of this intention is to pay particular attention to your performance.

Most of my work is done online. I meet with clients at the start of their journey for a consultation and body composition measurement, and then communicate with clients via email and *WhatsApp*. Why? Because they live busy and hectic lives. From balancing work, family, kids, the gym, and social activities, many of my clients barely have time to come in for a thirty-minute follow-up! Also bear in mind things like rush hour and general traffic, so meeting online makes a lot of sense.

But why is this relevant? Because, given the fast-paced and hectic world we live in today, we need foods and fluids to perform. I don't mean exercise performance only; I'm alluding to work performance, as well.

Whether you are an employee or a student at a university, healthy nutrition will significantly increase your performance. If you have a day full of meetings, presentations to give, tasks and deadlines, coursework, exams, etc.... you need to properly fuel your brain to improve things like focus, concentration, decision-making, and problem-solving.

Based on my experience working with clients, I've found that many clients tend to forget about eating and drinking throughout the day because they're so consumed with work. If they do eat, they'll usually choose unhealthy snack options like cookies, sweets, biscuits, and chocolate.

If you're the type of person who tends to skips meals because of stress, anxiety, and other emotions that stem from work and/or university, yet you still manage to perform well, imagine what your performance would be like if you were to eat more regularly, eat nutrient-dense food, and stay hydrated throughout the day.

I always like to use the analogy of a car and petrol when explaining the benefits of nutrition on the mind and body. A car needs petrol to run smoothly. Fill up a car with low-quality petrol, and it won't drive as efficiently or for such a long period of time. Fill up a car with high-quality petrol, and the car will drive smoother and for long distances.

Think about foods and fluids in the same way. If you provide your body (car) with nutrient dense foods (petrol), you will think more clearly and perform better at work and the gym. Skip meals or eat unhealthy foods, and you won't provide your body with the nutrients needed to boost mental performance.

It's imperative that, during stressful times, you put the time and effort into eating healthy food to boost performance. After all, don't associate food with only the body.

Think of food for the mind. Indeed, our brain uses food for energy—particularly glucose, which results from the digestion of carbohydrates. Provide your body with healthy and nutritious food, and you'll boost mental performance. You'll be able to think more clearly throughout the day, and also boost energy, focus, and concentration to allow you to handle tasks more efficiently and go about your day with more energy. All of which will improve your mood! And of course, the better our moods are, the happier we are as individuals.

Feed your brain with nutrient dense foods and experience the many benefits that come along with this practice.

Here are some foods to increase brain power:

- Oily fish (i.e. salmon)
- Nuts
- Avocado
- Turmeric
- Mixed berries
- Dark chocolate
- Coffee

Stay Hydrated

Hydration plays a huge role in the mind, as well. As with healthy food, staying hydrated with water can enhance decision making, improve problem-solving abilities, and transport oxygen and nutrients to the brain. It can even control hunger and appetite levels.

Sometimes you may feel hungry, but that doesn't necessarily mean you are in need of food. It may very well be dehydration.

Oftentimes, people forget to drink water throughout the day, again because of being too consumed with work and studying. Just as I said to prioritize food during stressful and busy situations, it's equally important to prioritize hydration.

Here are some tips to drink more water during the day:

- Drink 1-2 glasses with every main meal and snack.

- Eat more fruits and vegetables to also hydrate through foods.

- Drink soup.

- Take water wherever you go. Put it in your backpack, purse, or on your office desk.

- Buy a water bottle to help track how much water you drink. Set daily targets for how many times you want to fill up and drink the contents of your water bottle.

- Add flavor for taste. Funny enough, some people don't drink enough water because they don't like the taste. To make it more interesting and enjoyable, add some lemon or orange slices for a bit of flavor to promote drinking more water.

- Add a little salt to your food. Salt can help retain water in the body, but also triggers thirst mechanisms to drink more water.

Chapter 25
Meditation And Nutrition

*"Meditation is offering your genuine presence
to yourself in every moment."*

Terri Guillemets

I've mentioned meditation several times now through-out this book, and for a reason. Why? Because meditation is such a powerful tool to work on mindfulness, and as I already mentioned, mindfulness can significantly help with living a healthier lifestyle. While meditation can improve many aspects of your life, it can directly and indirectly affect your eating habits and behavior.

In this day and age, it's so easy to get consumed by everything that goes on around you. When that happens, you can end up feeling really stressed, anxious, and frustrated, which then takes you away from living in the moment. What happens a lot during these situations? Stress or emotional eating. What do we usually seek during these situations? Comfort. And what is one way to provide comfort? Food. And what foods are usually the ones that provide us with comfort? Fried foods, chocolate, and sweets. Basically, unhealthy foods.

Meditation is the practice of coming back to life. It helps train your mind to be more aware and take control of your emotions, thoughts, and feelings. Especially in this fast-paced and hectic world we live in, meditation can help bring you back to Earth and understand the space you're in.

Meditation is a beautiful practice, which I urge a lot of people to practice. Why? Because there are a lot of benefits that come with it:

1. Improving Self-Awareness

Meditation allows you to live in the present moment. Being self-aware can increase your ability to take control of your emotions and allow you to redirect your thoughts to have a clearer mind. All of which can help you with emotional eating and allow you to eat healthier.

2. Decreasing Anxiety

Do you feel anxious at work sometimes? Perhaps you feel anxious at home? In all cases, meditation can help decrease feelings of anxiety, whether socially or work related.

3. Reducing Stress

We all experience stress during the day in some form or another. Stress increases levels of cortisol, a stress hormone which can cause unwanted side effects.

Meditation helps reduce stress and make you feel calm and peaceful throughout the day, allowing you to approach food in a healthy manner.

4. Increasing Focus And Concentration

Believe it or not, meditation can actually help you stay more focused because it helps improve self-awareness. Practicing meditation keeps you in control, which can improve your cognitive function at work, university, or in any activity that you go about throughout the day. By staying focused in everyday life, you can also stay focused on living a healthy lifestyle by consistently eating well and exercising.

You may be thinking to yourself, *Why are you talking about meditation in a book that's predominantly about nutrition?* Well, that's because meditation is arguably the best way to *fill your mind* and to make you more aware of what you eat. The direct effects of meditation can have indirect effects on your nutrition—increasing your food awareness, and helping you eat more slowly and chew more.

Basically, it helps with everything covered in discussing P*illar 3—Mindfulness.*

The benefits of meditation are vast.

These are just some of the things I've experienced myself and thought I'd share with you. Like anything else, meditation requires time and practice. Even if you start with five minutes of meditation per day, that's good enough. With time, you can start increasing the duration as you get better and better at it. I'm no expert, and there is still much more room for improvement in my case, but the positive experiences that come along with it are the motivation for me to keep practicing.

And, believe me, once you start feeling the same effects, you won't want to stop. Once you see positive changes in your eating habits, as well, you'll have much more encouragement to continue.

Chapter 26
Make A Healthy Lifestyle A Part Of You

*"Looking good and feeling good go hand in hand.
If you have a healthy lifestyle, your diet and nutrition
are set, and you're working out you're going to feel good."*

Jason Statham

Mindset. Belief. Mindfulness. Sacrifice. Habits. Everything is connected.

Leading a healthy lifestyle can seem complicated. But you already have everything you need to change your life from the inside out. All you need is the key to unlock the process.

Staying healthy is not about dieting. It's about changing your lifestyle for the better. It's about making wiser food choices, moving more, and stressing less. Everything is connected, and by changing one thing, you can create a positive chain reaction. Better food equals more energy. More energy equals better sleep. Better sleep equals healthier food decisions. It's a cycle!

The *Five Pillars* in this book are pillars for a reason. Think of these pillars like physical pillars keeping a building intact. Remove one pillar and the building becomes unstable. Keep removing the pillars, and eventually the building will collapse. It's the exact same thing when thinking about a transition into a healthy lifestyle. You need all five pillars to be truly successful. They all work in unison and they are all prerequisites to becoming a healthier and happier version of yourself.

The whole idea behind the pillars and this book is to eventually help you make a healthy lifestyle a part of you. Through the right mindset, self-belief, mindfulness, and sacrificing, you'll adopt healthier habits. Once you positively change your eating habits and behavior, you'll start to do the right things without thinking. Your brain will start to work in autopilot mode, but in a healthy way. Eventually, you'll find yourself automatically making the right choices not because you have to, but because you want to.

This is the point which I hope for you to reach—and reach it, you will!

Thankfully, through many years of practice, dedication, and commitment, I've been able to reach this point. I'm not living a healthy lifestyle because I want to show off to others that I'm healthy. I don't follow health trends.

I most certainly don't do it for show (being healthy to achieve a summer body, for example). I do it because I value and appreciate the feeling. I do it for the love of feeling and being healthy. For the feeling of increased self-confidence and being able to love my own self. For the increased energy and focus I get after working out and giving my body the right nutrients to perform at the best level possible, either at work or at the gym. I hate feeling lethargic, bloated, or guilty after eating unhealthy food. I just hate it. Thus, I keep chasing the feeling I get from being healthy, and I'm constantly rewarded for that pursuit.

It truly is a beautiful feeling once you reach the point of simply being healthy. It's something that will simply make-up who you are. It will be a part of you, and if it's missing, you'll most certainly feel it.

Whether it's skipping out on training, or going days or weeks by eating unhealthily and not being in your routine, you'll feel off. I'm telling you this based on my own experience as well as years of successfully training and work with clients.

But I think those who are really into living a healthy lifestyle also feel the same way—this isn't an isolated impression.

Take Kevin Hart, for example. In the same podcast I mentioned earlier, he was discussing with Joe Rogan his exercise habits and how he feels if he doesn't train.

Here's what he had to say:

Joe Rogan: So, your whole purpose is to keep your vitality up, keep your energy up?

Kevin Hart: If I don't do it, then there's a lag. I need to train. I'm so mentally invested now that if I don't do it, I feel like I've cheated myself in a day or a week that I've taken off. I feel like, 'Yo man, I'm not myself.' Because when I am doing it, I feel like I'm committed. I'm committed to constantly building and reshaping and molding – I'm working on me. So, when I am not working on me, I don't feel like my day that is supposed to be about me is starting off with the biggest bang. This is my advantage to starting off like nobody else.

I can most certainly relate to Kevin on this. If I miss a day of training, or shy away from my healthy eating habits and eat unhealthy foods, I just feel like I did something wrong. I don't feel like myself. Not feeling comfortable in your own skin is not a pleasant feeling, and so that's why I keep making it a point to live a healthy lifestyle. After all, it's who I am and what makes me feel the happiest and most comfortable. This is my motivation to continue doing what I do.

With that said, living healthy is a combination of everything that makes you human; mind, body, and soul. Before you fill your plate, you need to fill your mind—making room for the mindset you need to produce long-term results.

Stay healthy. Stay focused. Stay connected.

Chapter 27
You Know Yourself Best

*"Don't be confused between what people say you are
and who you know you are."*

Oprah Winfrey

Dairy-free. Gluten-free. Sugar-free. High fat. Low carb. Intermittent fasting. Fasted cardio. High-intensity exercise. Crossfit. Yoga.

What's the best way to eat? What's the best workout to do? What's the best diet?

Do I have the answers for you? Yes, I do for my clients. But at this distance, no. So, can I tell you what's the best way to do things? No. Why? Because maybe it won't work for you. Perhaps what works for me or someone else may not work for you.

At the end of the day, I can sit here and advise you on what you should and shouldn't do. The foods you should and shouldn't eat. But that's not the purpose of this book. The purpose here is to make you understand that living a healthy lifestyle doesn't start with going on a diet or signing up for classes at a gym. Yes, that's part of a healthy lifestyle, but in my opinion—professional and personal—that shouldn't be your first thought.

Looking within (by focusing on the *Five Pillars*), understanding yourself, engaging in self-reflection and criticism, knowing your why, and gaining self-awareness is what will take you from not living a healthy lifestyle to living one. All of this will make you understand what works best for you, and help you understand and listen to your body.

Even though I can advise you to do what would be best for you, based on the literature and science, at the end of the day, you know yourself. You know y*our body.*

As John Berardi, co-founder of Precision Nutrition, once said, "You are the expert on your own body."

Living a healthy lifestyle comes with a lot of trial and error. By experimenting with different foods and ways of eating, and training in different ways and at different times of the day, you'll eventually come to know what works best for you. And when it comes to whatever it is that will work best for you, stick with it!

The best diet, the best types of exercise, and the most effective way to living a healthy lifestyle is doing things and living in a way that works best for you. Doing things that suit your schedule, routine, and lifestyle. Things that you actually will stick to. This will help you stay consistent and committed for the long term.

Don't do anything you don't enjoy. Don't do anything you feel uncomfortable doing, or anything that just doesn't feel right. You most certainly don't want to feel like you have to go out of your way to do something or feel like it's a burden. Feelings like this eventually lead to dropping out of a program and going back to your old habits.

This is why I alluded to the fact that time and patience is key for a healthy lifestyle. The more time you devote to your journey, the more you'll be able to experiment with different things and be able to understand what exactly it is that works best for you.

You know yourself best.

Section 4

Final Strategies And Steps

Fill Your Mind Before You Fill Your Plate

Chapter 28
The 7 Principles Of A Healthy Lifestyle

I didn't change myself all at once.

The *Pillars* came sequentially, in just the way I discussed them in this book. One pillar led to the next. I needed to precede each pillar with another in order to proceed in my journey.

I have already discussed the *Five Pillars*, but along my journey, there were also some principles that I abided by which helped me stay calm and collected. Some principles have already been discussed and overlap with the pillars, but that's also part of the point here. You'll realize that there is a common theme when wanting to live a healthier lifestyle.

Not in any specific order, here are my seven principles of changing over to a healthy lifestyle:

1. Have The Right Mindset

Yes, this is one of the *Five Pillars*, and also a very important principle. I've already discussed how important it is to develop the right mindset. It's so important that it's both a pillar and a principal of mine.

2. Be Patient

I want to lose weight, NOW! The amount of times I hear this from my clients and people in general has been countless. I'm sorry to burst your bubble, but whatever goal you've set for yourself needs time. I've not only experienced it myself, but I'm also experiencing it in my current line of work.

It's those clients who are patient that see the rewards at the end of their time working with me. Please, be patient with your goals and give them as much time as they realistically require. Time is your best friend when trying to be a healthier version of yourself, so patience is key.

3. Put In The Work

You are in the driver's seat. It's you who will make the decisions for yourself and take charge, not anybody else. That being said, you have to put the work in. Don't wait and sit around for things to come to you. To be healthy, you need to go for it and chase the lifestyle. It won't automatically morph into you. You have to morph into it.

4. Commitment

I know it can be really tough to commit to something, especially a healthy lifestyle. When I first started to live a healthier lifestyle, the thought of transitioning into a new way of life and leaving my old one behind was quite scary, to say the least. The fact that I also knew it was going to be a long and tiring journey was also scary. However, if I wanted to see results, I had to commit.

5. Do What You Enjoy

All principals mentioned here are important, but I can't stress enough the magnitude of this one. If you want to commit to something, do something that you enjoy! When it comes to training, participate in some sort of physical activity that you enjoy doing. When it comes to nutrition, don't necessarily follow specific diets and place limitations on yourself. Eat foods that you enjoy eating while of course staying mindful of your food choices and decisions. Doing something you enjoy will keep you committed for a longer period of time and will minimize the risk of relapsing.

6. Have Fun

With enjoyment comes fun. Your journey needs to be a fun and exciting one. Again, this will make it all the more interesting for you and increase compliance and commitment to the lifestyle.

Being healthy doesn't mean locking yourself at home. Go out and enjoy your time with friends and family. Eat out at restaurants, order in, and visit friends and family and enjoy eating meals with them, too. Just try to be as mindful as possible in those situations. The bottom line, though, is to have fun and put yourself in situations that bring you joy.

7. Reward Yourself

If you've accomplished a smaller goal and taken another step towards the bigger goal, reward yourself! Whether this comes through positive self-talk or rewarding yourself with a meal or food that you love, the key is to recognize your achievements. Praise yourself and be proud of your work and effort.

Chapter 29
You Don't Have To Do It On Your Own

Your surroundings make a huge difference in your lifestyle. The people you surround yourself with and the environment you put yourself in can really make or break your attempt to become a healthier version of yourself.

I think one of the biggest reasons why I was able to start and sustain my transition into a healthier lifestyle was related to my surroundings. When I told you about my *sick in the head phase,* I mentioned that it started in university, which was a big inspiration for me.

Seeing people jogging at 6am, collegiate athletes walking around campus, and even my own friends being dedicated to the gym, really helped me stay motivated throughout the process.

I think that if I'd started this journey back home in Kuwait, it would've been a far more difficult process. I probably wouldn't even have thought of starting this journey to begin with, in all honesty. Although there is much more awareness given to living a healthy lifestyle now in comparison to when I moved to the US, the society, culture, and traditions make it easier to move less and eat more. This just goes to show that you have to be aware of your surroundings, and understand how they can help or hinder you in your journey—make change where you can, and plan for the obstacles when it comes to everything else that doesn't work in your favor.

Motivational speaker Jim Rohn once said: *You are the average of the five people you spend the most time with.* And it's true.

Your people and environment are a determining factor in your overall ability to see and affect change. It's important that you surround yourself with people who are like-minded. People who will help support you throughout your journey and uplift your spirit during the good and bad times. It's tough to go about change all on your own, but it's even tougher to do so when you're in a difficult environment.

Friends and family are not your only means of support. There is absolutely nothing wrong with seeing a health coach or therapist. In fact, I'd highly encourage you to do so, especially if you think you lack the right mindset to get yourself going. You know, it's funny, but when people want to see change in their health, they always look towards a personal trainer or nutritionist first rather than looking inward, but that really is a first step.

As I've mentioned numerous times throughout this book, everything begins in the mind, and having the right mentality will set the tone for everything else.

Where I come from, seeing a therapist/psychologist is frowned upon. Or at least it's definitely kept secret. For some reason, people feel ashamed and embarrassed to see someone for their mental health. Getting support to grow and strengthen your own mental health is exactly the same thing as going to a gastroenterologist to strengthen your gut health.

Literally, it's the same thing! You're just working on a different part of your body.

So, if you're reading this and are one of those individuals who feel ashamed about talking to someone, or know of someone who may need help but feels embarrassed, please know that there is absolutely nothing wrong with seeking out a therapist or outside help.

You're only bettering yourself!

Chapter 30
Choosing A Nutritionist

Five Things To Look Out For
When Choosing A Nutritionist

Today, we're faced with so much information on the internet, and so many nutritionists on social media, that we're confused as to what's actually right for us. What should we eat? What should we avoid? Nutrition is becoming more and more complicated—much more than it should be!

I want to share with you my experience of working with other nutritionists as well as clients. I'm not here to brag or lash out against other nutritionists. This list can hopefully serve as a guide so that you'll know what to look for when seeking a nutritionist's help and guidance.

Here are five things to look out for:

1. Know Their Background

Fortunately, and unfortunately, so many certifications are available today, and this makes it easy for anyone and everyone to becoming a *certified* nutritionist. With that being said, it's so important to know the nutritionist you are dealing with. Ask them about their education, qualifications, and even experience working in the field.

I would recommend you go to someone who actually has a formal education in nutrition, dietetics, or a related field. That means having a Bachelors and/or Masters in the appropriate field. Your health lies in the hands of this person, so you want to make sure that he or she is qualified and credible!

2. Find Their Work

Look into the nutritionist you are working with and see if they have perhaps written any blogs, books, and/or published journal articles. If you can *Google* them and find their pieces of work, then you can tell the nutritionist is proactive in the field and actually doing his/her work with passion.

3. Observe Their Physique

You want to get advice from a nutritionist who actually *looks* like a nutritionist. The last thing you want is to get eating advice from someone who doesn't actually represent and define the advice and guidelines they give you.

Would you want to see a dentist with bad teeth?

4. They Should Practice What They Preach

Along the lines of that last point, it's so important to see nutritionists who stand by what they do and believe in what they do. Let me give you a hypothetical example: If you're seeing a sports nutritionist who doesn't work out and doesn't know what it feels like to train at varying intensities, is it a good idea to get sports nutrition advice from them? Some food for thought.

Let me give you another hypothetical example: If a nutritionist tells you one thing, but goes off behind the scenes and personally does another thing, you can tell they aren't really practicing what they preach. That's the bottom line: See a nutritionist who practices what they preach.

5. Evaluate Their Way Of Work

I have great respect for people in the field trying to help others become healthier versions of themselves. Providing value to society is a beautiful thing. With that said, though, be aware of who you choose and make sure the nutritionist you work with is qualified and credible when it comes to giving you health advice, guidance, and coaching.

Does the nutritionist show genuine care in your goal and change toward a healthier lifestyle? Are they creating a friendly relationship that's more than just a nutritionist-client relationship? Do they educate you along the way and make you understand why they are giving you certain advice, or why they structure their meal programs the way they do? If you answer no to any of these questions, you need to revisit your decision of seeing that nutritionist.

Four Red Flags That Indicate You Shouldn't Choose This Nutritionist

Having worked in the field of nutrition for a few years now, I've listened carefully to the words and feedback of my clients, as well as people in general who've seen other nutritionists.

Unfortunately, I've heard plenty of stories regarding mistakes made when seeking a nutritionist, which has led people to feel frustrated about not reaching their goals and feeling and looking the way they want to be.

Again, I do not intend this section to be a means of lashing out against any other nutritionist in the field. This list should simply serve as a guide for you when it comes to being aware of such pitfalls, to then not repeat the same mistakes as others!

1. Don't Mistake The Number Of Social Media Followers For Credibility

Some people may see a nutritionist because of their big social media following. Seeking a nutritionist is not a numbers game. It's not about how many followers they have. They may just have the right personality and charisma on social media, but this may not necessarily translate into being a good nutritionist.

Don't let the number of followers get in your way when making choices of who to see!

2. Weight Loss

Just because a nutritionist lost a ton of weight doesn't make them legitimate. *What worked for them may not work for you.* And what works for you may not work for others! Don't judge nutritionists by their own weight loss journey.

3. Education

Make sure the nutritionist you see is actually qualified and credible through formal education in nutrition or a similar field—not just through a certification.

You want to make sure the person you see has many years of studying and learning in the field. This doesn't necessarily entail getting a certification over a few months, which many people can do.

4. One Size Fits All

As a nutritionist, it can be very tempting to create standardized programs. It saves a lot of time and it can drive more sales to simply print a sheet of paper and hand it out to everyone. This is a big red flag.

Nutrition should be very individualized to each person. Everyone has a different body type and genetic make-up. People like different foods and also respond differently to various foods.

So, the next time you work with a nutritionist, make sure their work is customized to you.

Chapter 31
Considering The Lifestyle Change

Before you want to make change, you have to change yourself. This comes with a lot of introspection. I'm not going to sit here and write this book telling you how pleasant and easy it is to do that. It can be quite emotionally and mentally draining, in fact. But hey, if it was easy, then we would all be the healthiest and fittest people, right? It's all part and parcel of making a change. If after reading this book you feel more motivated and inspired to get started and begin the change process, you now know where to start—in your mind.

The thing is, though, I know it may be very difficult for you to talk to someone about your issues, or simply seek out guidance and help. To think of speaking to someone, let alone having someone tell you what to do, can be quite scary, I know. Even though you've confirmed to yourself that there's something you need to change, whether it's the way you look or feel physically and/or mentally, or some aspect of your lifestyle in general, the thought of this can cause you not to take any action at all.

Whether this is the case or not, I urge you to look inside yourself for help first.

So, how do you start?

First, you really have to spend a lot of time in self-reflection. Look at the many aspects of your life and consider some things:

- How do you currently feel about yourself? The way you look?
- How do you want to look and feel?
- If you have a family, do you want to be a role model to your kids and grandkids?
- Maybe you want to look good in front of your wife or husband?
- Do you want to perform well at your job? Perhaps get the salary raise or promotion you've always longed for?
- What about exercise? Do you want to be able to train in a specific way, achieve a certain exercise movement, or simply hit your personal best records?
- Do you just want to feel good while going about your daily activities (i.e. walking up the stairs without feeling tired)?
- Are you feeling anxious, depressed, or stressed? Do you want to have a calmer and more positive outlook on life?

Honestly, there are so many things to consider when deciding to make change. It's very subjective, though, and you have to figure out what's suitable for you and your lifestyle, as well as what means the most to you and what you want to prioritize.

Who are you now and who do you want to be—and why?

That's what I asked myself at the early onset of my change process, and it's what you have to ask yourself now. Other than self-reflection, you can start taking the initiatives to look elsewhere for help while still being in control of your own actions and decisions:

- Self-talk. Literally, talk to yourself, whether out loud or inside your head (this might sound crazy, but it really does work!).

- Listen to podcasts.

- Read self-help/guidance books or listen to audio books during your commute to and from work.

- Spend time alone to further self-reflect.

- Meditate.

- Attend workshops.

- Go on a retreat (if you can go alone, that would be even better).

- Surround yourself with people who motivate and inspire you.

Visualization

According to the Oxford Dictionary, visualization is the *formation of a mental image of something.*

This played a huge role in my journey, and still plays an important role for me today.

When I first read into visualization, I used to think to myself how lame this change technique seemed. Some of you reading this might think the same, too.

I remember that one day I decided to read *The 7 Habits of Highly Effective People* by Stephen Covey. It wasn't until after I read this book and actually started to engage in *Habit 2* that I realized how truly powerful visualization could be.

Habit 2 refers to *beginning with the end in mind:*

"Habit 2 is based on imagination--the ability to envision in your mind what you cannot at present see with your eyes. It is based on the principle that all things are created twice. There is a mental (first) creation, and a physical (second) creation. The physical creation follows the mental, just as a building follows a blueprint. If you don't make a conscious effort to visualize who you are and what you want in life, then you empower other people and circumstances to shape you and your life by default. It's about connecting again with your own uniqueness and then defining the personal, moral, and ethical guidelines within which you can most happily express and fulfill yourself.

Begin with the End in Mind means to begin each day, task, or project with a clear vision of your desired direction and destination, and then continue by flexing your proactive muscles to make things happen.

One of the best ways to incorporate *Habit 2* into your life is to develop a *Personal Mission Statement.* It focuses on what you want to be and do. It is your plan for success. It reaffirms who you are, puts your goals in focus, and moves your ideas into the real world. Your mission statement makes you the leader of your own life. You create your own destiny and secure the future you envision."

Now, that's deep.

During university, whether I was living in a dorm or an apartment, I used to always have pictures of people who motivated and inspired me. Not only on the wall, but even as my wallpaper on both my phone and laptop! These people were actually my role models.

It started off with two individuals who I mentioned already, Cristiano Ronaldo and Kobe Bryant. My third role model, I discovered in 2010—Kendrick Lamar, the greatest rapper of today.

Why make their pictures the wallpaper for my phone and laptop? Because these were two devices that I used not only on a daily basis, but multiple times a day. So even though I wasn't surrounded by my idols, the fact that I saw them on my wallpaper multiple times a day, every day, kept me grounded and reminded me of the person I wanted to be in my own life. Of course, my living situation was key, too. That's where I spent most of my time, so having pictures on the wall also served as a daily reminder and further motivation.

Earlier in the book, I mentioned how it can be very helpful to have a role model to provide the motivation and inspiration you need to keep you going. I was fortunate enough to actually find my role models without struggle, but for you, this might not be the case. You can still do something similar, though—for example, finding a picture of someone who has the body you're trying to achieve and work towards. Sometimes, I'd change up the wallpaper on my devices and show a quote or a word that really resonated with me.

One of them was, of course, *BELIEVE*. This word is currently on my wall, with another quote, as well: *Strive for greatness.*

Visualization doesn't stop here, though. Visualization can purely be in the mind. You don't need to necessarily have pictures in front of you (although I think this is a really helpful technique). Scientists have referred to motivational generally-mastery imagery as a good way to help you towards your goals. This is basically envisioning you climbing up that hill, or pushing through a workout, or achieving a certain exercise that you have been working on for a long time. Not only does this technique help you achieve your goals, but it can remove any feeling of doubt and fear.

You also have a visualization technique known as *mental imagery.* According to *The Sandford Encyclopedia of Philosophy,* mental imagery is referred to as *visualizing, seeing in the mind's eye, hearing in the head,* and/or *imagining the feel of.*

Mental imagery resembles *perceptual experience, but occurs in the absence of the appropriate external stimuli.*

Why is this relevant?

Because it can actually help people eat healthier. Believe it or not, individuals have used this technique to increase their intake of fruits and vegetables. By simply visualizing themselves eating the fruit or vegetable, touching it, smelling it, and eating from it, this method helped them achieve their goal of increasing their consumption of such foods.

Aside from the technique of using images as a way to engrain a certain vision or goal in my mind, I've used (and still do use) mental imagery in a gym setting. As an avid calisthenics' trainer, I do engage in things like handstands and hand-stand push-ups.

Many times, I've actually stood back, closed my eyes, and visualized myself going through the handstand process successfully. Believe you, me, it works!

Mental imagery has really helped me through my calisthenics journey, and while I would say my progress is mostly related to continual practice, this definitely played a part in achieving my training goals.

Whether you have a nutrition or training goal in mind, if are willing to do things on your own, spend some time implementing visualization techniques. It will help you overcome feelings of doubt and fear, acquire new skills, and you accelerate towards your goals.

Chapter 32
Conclusion

As an inspired and motivated individual, I believe it is only necessary to help transform the lives of others ... to help them find their own path to greatness—inside and out.

Health and fitness are my life. This pursuit has changed me as an individual. It has been the driving force to being the best I can be. Not only has my healthy lifestyle journey taught me so much about myself, but it taught me so much about life. The negative emotions and struggles helped me cope with the frustrating and stressful moments in life. The positive and joyful moments motivated me to continue working towards being the best I can be to continually experience those moments, while always reminding me to enjoy these moments and embrace them.

The biggest challenge I face as a nutritionist is getting people to believe in the power of healthy nutrition. Everyone knows that eating a chocolate bar or devouring a *Big Mac* will send your organs crying out for help. What they don't know is how their quality of life can significantly improve when they sprinkle their diet with clean, unprocessed, and healthy food, exercising on a regular basis and of course developing a positive mindset.

In 2017, I founded the nutrition consultancy firm known as *Believe Nutrition*. The name *Believe Nutrition* stems from the backdrop of my wanting to help people believe in the powerful effects nutrition has on both the mind and body. I want to help people believe in the incredibly empowering effects of a healthy lifestyle, from having the right mindset to well-balanced nutrition and daily exercise. I want to instill a desire in people to consistently lead a sustainable life full of health and happiness. Most importantly, I want to instill the belief of one's own power to bring about change.

And it all starts with knowledge.

Perhaps you have the courage and confidence to finally work with someone. After all, there's absolutely nothing wrong with turning to someone for help and getting some form of support. There are only so many books you can read and podcasts you can listen to before, at some point, you may find yourself wanting some professional help, and that's completely fine. I encourage you to find some sort of social support anyway, whether it's finding a coach, mentors, or simply turning to your family and friends.

Through my experiences, both personally and professionally, I've come to a point in my life where I can confidently coach people to help them become a healthier and better version of themselves.

Using a simple, informed, and science-based approach, I help guide clients in taking action to shape their body, enhance their nutrition, and commit to a lifestyle that works best for them. Whether they're tied up at work or at home, I'll guide them in learning the tools they need to approach nutrition, fitness, and mindful eating with confidence.

My current line of work revolves around approaching a healthy lifestyle holistically.

Focusing on nutrition, training, and health coaching (mindset) as a whole. In order for you to reach your goal, a holistic approach needs to be found.

With my clients, I create individualized nutrition programs to suit their lifestyle, exercise abilities/routines, and any food dislikes, allergies, and/or intolerances. Coupled with nutrition are also individualized training programs to help bridge the two together. After all, to get the best out of your training, a sound nutrition program must be put in place. To further accelerate you towards your nutrition and body goals, exercise is highly recommended, too. The two go hand in hand. Taking all of these elements into consideration, I've also developed a habit-based curriculum that focuses not only on behavioral change, but also on improving eating habits, as well. For example, mindful eating and others that I've mentioned in Chapter 18.

I don't believe in diets. Nor do I believe in taking control of my clients' decisions and lifestyles. I'm here to coach my clients into living a healthier lifestyle through their own way of being. It's really hard to change your own self, and even harder to change other people. That's why I work in a collaborative fashion with my clients, and in such a way that allows them to come up with solutions themselves. Solutions that they think will fit into their lifestyle nicely and not act as a barrier or burden to change.

I can easily provide textbook guidelines and advice to my clients. Creating a meal plan is also easy. But that's not the only thing to be considered. I really need to consider my clients' lifestyle, social support, mentality, emotions, and other aspects of life to get the best out of them. To help them become a healthier and happier version of themselves.

Because, after all, that is my mission.

More importantly, I work in a way that takes into account real-life situations. I can easily provide *perfect* nutrition or training programs to my clients. The thing is, we don't live in a p*erfect* world, and nor are we *perfect* ourselves. Life today presents us with many challenges.

Unfortunately, we live in a fast-paced and hectic world. We experience stress from work, growing responsibilities from family and friends, social events, peer pressure, and so many other factors that can scare us away from trying to lead a healthier lifestyle. That said, I factor this into the equation and try to accommodate my clients' lifestyle to the utmost degree in order to make sure they go through the process of change within their own realm and capabilities. It's one thing to take theory into practice, and another to take that practice and apply it to real life situations.

If you work with me, I'll do the best I can to do just that and help you spring to change, mentally and physically.

Our bodies are beautifully complex creations. To be able to listen, to understand and to love your body, is an unparalleled feeling. Through my work, I aim to help change not just your physical well-being, but also your mental well-being. I will teach you how to shape your body and enhance your nutrition and exercise routines to get the results you've always wanted.

Your body is a work of art. Let me help you beautifully sculpt it and embrace the feeling of being healthy.

References

- Covey. S (1989). *The 7 Habits of Highly Effective People.* Franklin Covey

- Covey, S. (2014). *The 7 Habits of Highly Effective Teens: The Ultimate Teenage Success* Guide. New York, NY. Simon and Schuster

- Dweck, C.S. PhD (2006). *Mindset: The New Psychology Of Success.* Ballantine Books.

- Hassad. C. & McKenzie. S. (2012). *Mindfulness For Life.* Robinson.

- Prochchaska. J.O, Norcross J.C and DiClemente C.C. (1994). *Changing For Good.* Collins Living.

- Sinek, Simon. (2009). *Start With Why: How Great Leaders Inspire Everyone to Take Action.* New York, NY. Portfolio.

About Faisal Alshawa

Faisal has always been passionate about health and fitness. As a child, he stayed active and played various sports. In 2008, Faisal moved to the US to study Kinesi -ology at the University of Maryland, College Park. After completing his under- graduate degree, he went on to attain a Masters' degree in Sports and Exercise 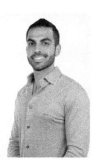 Science at Loughborough University. Faisal moved to Doha, Qatar after graduation and was designated as a sports nutritionist for the *U23 Qatar National Olympic Football Team.* During this time, he was also assigned to administer sports nutrition services to the *U19 Qatar National Football Team,* athletes in track and field, squash, and table tennis.

His experience working in various sports, as well as competitive and recreational athletes, led Faisal to start *Believe Nutrition* consultancy in June of 2017.

Believe Nutrition helps individuals and all levels of athletes, from beginner to professional, to believe in the power of nutrition. As the founder of *Believe Nutrition,* Faisal wants to instill a positive change in peoples' lives through a holistic approach, which focuses on the mind, body and soul. Faisal does not want to help people for the short-term; rather, he strives to impart a passion for health on anyone he works with to ensure they become the best version of themselves, for the long-term. This is why *Believe Nutrition* was created.

How To Get In Touch

If you'd like to know more about me and *Believe Nutrition*, you can follow me on *Instagram* and *Facebook* and visit our website where you will have access to blogs and be able to book a consultation to get started on your healthy lifestyle journey!

Facebook/Instagram: *@believenutrition*

Website: *www.believenutrition.net*

Fill Your Mind Before You Fill Your Plate